Calm Your Mind
&
Warm Your Heart

Through the Ups and Downs of Cancer

Real Voices and Techniques to Support You

Dr. Catherine Phillips

Detselig Enterprises Ltd.
Calgary, Alberta

Library and Archives Canada Cataloguing in Publication

Phillips, Catherine, 1951-
    Calm your mind & warm your heart : through the ups and
downs of cancer / Catherine Phillips.
ISBN 978-1-55059-414-0
    1. Cancer–Patients–Psychology. 2. Cancer–Psychological
aspects. 3. Mind and body. 4. Self-care, Health. 5. Mental
healing. I. Title. II. Title: Calm your mind and warm your
heart.
RC262.P45 2011   616.99'4   C2011-906873-7

Detselig Enterprises Ltd
210, 1220 Kensington Rd NW
Calgary, Alberta
T2N 3P5

DETSELIG
ENTERPRISES LTD
Calgary, Alberta, Canada

www.temerondetselig.com
Ph. 403-283-0900
fax. 403-283-6947
email:
temeron@telusplanet.net

Detselig Enterprises Ltd. acknowledges the financial support of the
Government of Canada through the Canada
Books Program for our publishing program.   Canadä

Also acknowledged is the financial assistance of the Alberta
Multimedia Development fund of the Government of Alberta, for the
support of our publishing program.

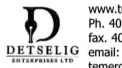

ISBN 978-1-55059-414-0   Printed in Canada
E-pub ISBN 978-1-55059-431-7

Dedication

This book is dedicated to all the cancer patients and family members whose voices grace these pages. They have contributed far more than the material for this work. They illuminate the vary finest in our human spirit: both the pain and vulnerability of the thin line we all walk at times to find meaning and purpose amidst crisis and our capacity for peace and warm heartedness along the way. Their stories are our stories, at times sad and despairing, at other times, joyful and reaffirming of living life fully and meaningfully. Their lived experience pulses through the ups and downs of these pages, bringing a message of comfort and hope. It has been a privilege and an honor to work with them and to learn from their example.

The names and some circumstances of patients and family members described in this book have been changed to preserve their confidentiality.

To Marilyn, regards with warm

Cathy

Acknowledgments

This book would not have been possible without the support and guidance of several key people. First and foremost I would like to thank Dr. Alastair Cunningham, who started the Healing Journey program. His innovative vision, enthusiasm, and scientific rigor changed and developed the program for over 25 years into its present form. He mentored many clinicians and researchers along the way. I am grateful to be in their number. Fellow colleagues Dr. Claire Edmonds and Dr. Judy Gould also supported this book from the outset, providing key feedback at every point in the process. It was wonderful to know I could always turn to them for support, guidance and humor. Claire merits particular recognition as the co-leader of the year long research group that furnished most of the material for this book. Her warm and inspired leadership did much to enable participants to explore and express their thoughts and feelings on the wide array of topics covered here. Her contribution to the book and to the program is profound.

The Healing Journey is a community of leaders, participants and volunteers and all have influenced the shape of this book. In addition to Alastair, Claire, and Judy, I have had the pleasure of working closely with Ann Hampson, Roy Robertson, Jane Yager Thomas, Jean Jackson, Rachel Kampf, Dr. Kim Watson, Kathy Feher and many others in Healing Journey programs. Jan Ferguson has brought extraordinary care, warmth and enthusiasm to her role as co-ordinator of the program for over 15 years. In recent years, the Healing Journey Program has found a permanent home in Wellspring centres across Canada. Wellspring has been a vital life force and partner, fostering and supporting development, leadership training and wider accessibility to the program.

I am also grateful to many family members and friends who read drafts and gave helpful feedback. In particular, Barrie Barrell provided support and wise guidance. Finally, I tip my hat to my old friend, Dudleigh Coyle, who encounters most everything with a warm heart and the conviction: "It's all good."

Table of Contents

Introduction
Is this Book for You?

This book is about finding comfort, hope and healing no matter what you face in the course of cancer. And whether you are a cancer patient yourself or a partner, relative, or friend of someone living with cancer, this book has been written with you in mind.

The goal of the book is to help you calm your thoughts, warm your heart and find comfort on both good days and bad days – at times when things are going well and at times when the outlook looks and feels bleak. There are two important ways the book attempts to achieve this. Firstly it will teach you techniques and strategies to manage your worries and fears and warm and open your heart. Secondly and equally important, the book tells stories of people like yourself – cancer patients and their loved ones documenting what it was like for them to go through their ups and downs and how they dealt with the challenges and opportunities along the way.

To write this book, I'm drawing on my experience as a psychologist with a special interest in cancer care in both clinical and research settings. As a clinician, I've had the privilege of working closely with cancer patients teaching coping skills, leading support groups and practising as an individual therapist. I have heard many stories and observed a wide range of responses to the challenges cancer brings to patients and their families. As a researcher, I've been part of a team led by Dr. Alastair Cunningham at the Princess Margaret Hospital in Toronto, studying the impact of psychological self-help work on patients attending our Healing Journey program. The program, designed to help people cope more effectively with illness, has an extensive research archive consisting of patients' first-hand accounts of their lived experiences. The majority of quotes in this book are drawn from this rich archive.

Often our research team would sit around the conference table to try to distill our experience into one sentence. What is healing? If we could put everything we had observed and learned into one sentence, what would that sentence be? We tossed about ideas, but the complexity of the subject and the diversity of experience didn't seem to lend itself to one definitive statement.

Then, a few years ago, I attended a series of teachings given by the Dalai Lama in Toronto. On the last day of the conference, the Dalai Lama responded to questions posed by participants. One of the questions was "How can I cure myself of my disease?" I listened very carefully to the answer.

The Dalai Lama replied, "The single most important thing you can do for healing . . ." He paused momentarily. He wanted to clarify that by healing, he meant not only physical healing of the body, but also emotional and spiritual healing as well. He repeated, "The single most important thing you can do for healing is to cultivate a warm heart."

"That's it!" I thought. One sentence that holds everything I have learned. Had I not worked closely for many years with cancer patients as a researcher and as a clinician, I probably would have dismissed this as a warm fuzzy notion. But experience has taught me to recognize the wisdom of these words. It is this wisdom that I hope to pass on to you through the stories of the people I have worked with and the techniques and strategies they have employed to calm their minds and warm their hearts.

If I succeed in my goals for this book you will find sustenance here both from the real words and stories of people like yourself and from learning new and effective techniques to help you live more peacefully. Chapters one to three focus on the troubled mind and how to calm it; chapters four to six on the troubled heart and how to warm it; chapter seven is for caregivers – the partners, family members and friends who support cancer patients; and chapter eight addresses the special challenges of living with advanced cancer.

Wherever you are on your cancer journey, there is always hope. If you are newly diagnosed, or have lived with cancer for many years; if you are the partner or friend of someone living with cancer; if your cancer is contained or if your cancer has spread; if your spirits are buoyant or if you're feeling tired, bleak and alone, there is hope. There is a place of opening from whatever point you are at.

My wish is that this book becomes like a trusted companion – a good friend you can turn to for whatever it is you need in the moment – whether it be inspiration, guidance, comfort, or a caring witness on those days when nothing seems to help or work. Even if I fail in this mission, I take comfort in my belief that the failure is mine and not a failure of the central truth this book attempts to convey: There is always hope; you are not alone; there are ways you can help yourself. And the surest way to find hope, comfort, and healing is to cultivate a calm mind and a warm heart.

One
The Troubled Mind

Quit trying to scare me

Those first words "You have cancer" strike like an electric jolt to your system. Whether the words are directed to you or someone you care about, the impact is often immediate – body tenses, mind whirls and spirit sags. How can this be happening? It doesn't seem real. Part of you refuses to believe it; the other part anticipates the worst. While people vary in their responses, more often than not, those first few days feel like a roller coaster. Here's how one woman described it:

> My first thoughts when I found out that I had breast cancer, just after surgery, were that somehow I would get through this and recover. I thought "I can deal with this." In the days that followed I experienced increasing fear, as I waited for the test results to determine how serious my cancer was. I was frightened in the hospital when nurses came to take me for further tests like bone and liver scans. They didn't give me an overview of what happens after an initial cancer diagnosis, and the tests led me to think the cancer might have spread. My husband and I went into a kind of shocked state once I got home – alternating between optimistic "pep talks" and crying about our worst fears.

When life suddenly feels like a roller coaster, there is not much you can do but hold on for the ride. Going up, there's an upbeat feeling: "I can deal with this. I can beat this thing. I will be back to my old self and my old life in no time." Going down, there's a panicky feeling: "What if . . . What if . . . What if . . ."

The "what ifs" vary from person to person and they present in different orders of importance. But the panicky feeling is the same. What if treatment doesn't work? What if I lose my job? What if I lose my looks? What if I leave my children? My partner? My parents? What if my friends and family fall away? What if I'm in pain? What if I can no longer do the things I love to do or be the person I want to be?

As a psychologist working with cancer patients and their families, I hear many stories of turmoil following diagnosis and the image of a roller coaster comes up frequently in descriptions of that time. While these stories always touch me, they no longer surprise me. But I was surprised by Sarah's roller coaster story.

Sarah is a single woman in her thirties with a demanding job and a busy life. When she learned she had breast cancer, her first thought was, "This can't be right." Her second thought was, "I must go on a roller coaster." While most people use the metaphor of a roller coaster to describe the ups and downs, Sarah used one literally. The very thought of a roller coaster filled her with terror. "That's why I had to do it," she told our support group.

It was a first session of an eight week breast cancer group at Wellspring, a community resource centre for people living with cancer and for their families. There are several Wellsprings in the Toronto area and across Canada and this particular group was meeting in the downtown Toronto location. Outside, the first signs of winter were setting in – grey skies and a sudden nip in the air. Inside it was warm and inviting as Wellspring makes a point of extending warmth and welcome to all who pass through its doors. Even with that welcome, first sessions tend to have an uncertain edge. People don't know what to expect. Naturally many are feeling a little apprehensive. They may be wondering, "Is this going to help me? Will I fit in here? What is the point of this?"

One of the major benefits of a support group is the shared experience of the membership. There is a sense of being heard, understood and cared for. The comments given most often are "I'm no longer alone" and "No one can understand what it is like to live with cancer as well as someone going through the same thing." Members also value the exchange of information and support about treatments and symptoms and how to deal with their thoughts and feelings about cancer and the impact it is having on their families, friends, work and all other aspects of their lives. But there is also the concern that hearing the stories of others may bring them down or awaken or intensify their own fears. Some are concerned that going to a group is "dwelling on the illness" instead of "getting on with life."

My role as facilitator is to foster a safe and comfortable environment for everyone in the room. This is especially important at the outset of a new group. I describe the benefits of support groups but I also acknowledge that it is sometimes hard to hear stories of others and it is not uncommon to feel anxious and unsettled in the first few sessions. Over time these feelings usually settle as members get to know one another and feel safe and comfortable with the group setting. Once that trust is there, the group can hold all the stories – stories of times when things are going well and stories of times when things are not going as well, feelings of peace and ease and feelings of distress and struggle. A large part of the first session is getting to know one another. People introduce themselves in whatever way feels comfortable for them. Usually they talk about their cancer, but not always. Sarah's introduction certainly caught the group's attention.

"I just had to do it" she said. "I had to go on that roller coaster. I thought if I can conquer this fear, I can conquer anything." Around the room, people looked uncertain. I sensed the various tensions that often accompany a first session. Some of the members looked stunned by what they heard; others enthralled. Then, tension broke as one woman laughed heartily. "You go, girl!" A ripple of laughter started and then rolled around the room like a wave. Everyone joined in. We laughed because it was an unusual story: we did not expect it. We laughed because the story cut through the awkwardness of introductions and immediately connected us as a group. We laughed because it felt good to laugh. And we laughed because suddenly in front of us was this stark and powerful truth – cancer is frightening.

Fear: The Silent Stalker

Fear is the silent stalker that follows a cancer diagnosis. Fear is the f word that is often repressed because of the havoc it might cause if given voice. Sarah named the stalker and fought it head on. Our very own heroine had gone out to slay the dragon. We applauded her. We bonded quickly as a group. The door had been opened to talk about fear.

Eleanor Roosevelt said, "We gain strength, and courage, and confidence by each experience in which we really stop to look fear in the face. We must do that which we think we cannot." She could have been talking to Sarah. Sarah felt intuitively that by facing her fear of roller coasters she would gain strength, courage and confidence to face her cancer experience. By telling her story to the group, she helped lay the foundation for the web of support and community that weaves a group together in solidarity against the ravages of that silent stalker – fear. Suddenly it was easier for others to talk about what was most on their minds, but most frightening to say. Simply to name it can come as a relief, "I'm frightened." Others nodded their heads. They knew. They were frightened too.

When people can't talk about their fears, often it is because they don't want to "give into them." They worry that giving attention to these frightening thoughts will make things worse. Sometimes superstitious thought underlies the need to keep fears in tight rein. The superstition goes something like this: "If I acknowledge I'm frightened, I'm making it real. If I give voice to my fears then they will come true. If I pretend I have no fear, maybe I can make the whole thing go away."

This strategy is appealing because it appears to work, at least for a while. When fearful thoughts arise, you push them away and carry on with your life, keeping very busy. The busier you are the better it is for keeping fears at bay. However, when you slow down or have a moment of quiet reflection, that niggling feeling that "all is not well" nags at you from the back of your mind or sometimes more stridently with unexpected emotional force. In the long run, facing fears, as Roosevelt wisely advised and Sarah intuitively felt, is the surest way to peace of mind.

But it is not a matter of all or nothing. There are times when dismissing fearful thoughts and getting on with your life makes a lot of sense and is exactly what you need to do. Ultimately, it is more useful to face fears than to dismiss them. But this does not mean that you must tackle your fears every time they come up. or live constantly with an awareness of your fears. In fact, learning to discharge the restless energy that comes with fearful thoughts and distracting yourself with other activities are some of the strategies presented in the next chapter for managing your thoughts.

So why face your fears at all? This is an important question. Perhaps neither Eleanor Roosevelt's quote, nor Sarah's intuitive example speak to you. Fears take away hope and stir turmoil in body, mind and spirit. So why face them if acknowledging them gives them voice and power? Why make yourself miserable?

This was the very question raised by a woman attending a Healing Journey program at Wellspring. We were about to do an exercise in which participants are led through a relaxation exercise and then invited to imagine their cancer, and if it feels right for them, to start a dialog with their image. As I was explaining the exercise, a woman in the front row, who I will call Susan, sighed audibly and asked, "What is the point of that? I don't want to imagine my cancer. It scares me. What if it looks huge? I didn't come here to be scared. I don't want to do this."

I agreed that the exercise could be scary and it was not very pleasant to come to a course and be scared. Also, some days are more difficult than others and on those days we may not feel comfortable doing such an exercise. Self-care is always important. Looking after your own comfort and wellbeing may mean choosing to sit out the exercise in the adjoining room or the library upstairs. Making such a choice was entirely fine.

I also thanked Susan for her courage in speaking out because there would be others in the room feeling the same way and it helped them and all of us to look at her important question, "What is the point of this? Why would I risk scaring myself by imagining my cancer?"

The group looked expectantly at me to supply the answer. But rather than quote Eleanor Roosevelt, or spout psychological theory, I turned to the group of twenty participants and asked them their thoughts on the subject. "What is the point of this? "

I do this routinely now with any group before a challenging exercise. I tell the story of Susan. Everyone can relate to her position – "I don't want to imagine my cancer. It scares me. What if it looks huge? I didn't come here to be scared. I don't want to do this."

A good discussion always ensues, sometimes with considerable emotion. There are varying viewpoints, but nonetheless, it amazes me that across many groups, over many years, a consensus of opinion emerges. "You do it because the fear is there." As one woman put it, "From the moment I first heard the word cancer, fear has been with me. It is not always foremost in my mind, but it is there. It's like I don't have any control over it.

Maybe these exercises will change that. Not the fear.I expect it will always be there in some form, but the way it takes hold."

Another woman's response to her fear speaks exactly to that point. She was in our long-term psychotherapy group which met for two and a half hours every week for a year, as part of a research study at Princess Margaret Hospital. She was a vibrant creative woman in her forties, who others in the group looked to for inspiration and wisdom. She was living with breast cancer which had spread to her lungs, liver and bones. One day when she felt in the grip of her fears, she turned to a stack of magazines that were lying around her house and started cutting out any image that related to how she was feeling. She brought the collage to the group to show to us.It was a bold, vivid, collection of images and colors. On the bottom she had written in big capital letters – QUIT TRYING TO SCARE ME.

While making her collage, she felt intensely engaged and alive. That, by itself, shifted her mood. But more importantly, afterwards she felt as if she had changed the dynamic of her fears. Instead of being a passive victim to them, she had summoned her own creative resources and actively responded with her own inner power. Hanging the collage in her kitchen was a constant reminder of both the darkness of the moment and her spirited response. The fears were still there, but she felt more powerful, more peaceful, more in control of her own responses.

That is the point. If we face our fears, instead of dismissing them, we get to know them better. We begin to see more effectively the hold they have on us. With greater awareness we also have more opportunities to summon new perspectives and connect with our own inner healing resources. We may not eliminate our fears, but we can work more actively with them and then choose to find affirmation, hope and meaning in ways that feel right to us. Such an achievement, as Eleanor Roosevelt says, brings strength, courage and confidence.

After hearing various points of view, Susan decided to try the exercise after all. When I asked her at the end of the session what the exercise had been like for her, she said it had been unexpectedly peaceful. She felt so profoundly relaxed during the initial part, that she stayed with that peaceful feeling and did not do the part of imagining her cancer. Instead she imagined a beautiful white light filling her entire being. "That sounds like just what you needed," I said. I encouraged her to use the same image at home during the week.

Susan's response highlights another important point – there is a place of opening from wherever we are and we can tackle our fears in our own time and in our own ways. There is no right way or wrong way of doing this. As we open to challenges presented to us, we can proceed gently in a way that "feels right" to us, as Susan's example illustrates.

So far we've been talking about the major fears that come with the territory of illness. The ones that scare us. But there are many other ways our minds are troubled by the experience of cancer and our habitual ways of looking at things. Our thoughts create our experience. If we have troubled thoughts, we have a restless and uneasy mind. Peace of mind is a long way off.

Finding Support In The Words Of Others

Remember, you're not alone in this. I'm hoping the stories and voices of others, like yourself, going through the same things, will provide some support for you, just as a cancer support group does for its members. From years of working with cancer patients, I have learned many worries are commonly shared. In fact, first time participants in a support group often remark at the end of the session, "It's been such a relief to know I'm not going mad. I thought I was the only one having these thoughts. Just hearing other people say the same things makes me feel not so alone."

When people say, "Oh, I wouldn't join a support group; I'm not a 'group' person; I like to handle things on my own," I know where they are coming from. I would have described myself in the same way before I had the privilege to work closely with people in groups. And while I certainly understand the need to figure things out for oneself and to manage on one's own, I have seen too many times the power of community to heal and soothe in both subtle and not so subtle ways to ever doubt the added benefits of joining a support group. And perhaps the most powerful benefit of all is the way a seasoned group can hold and support individuals through the toll of their fears and uncertainties.

That is what this chapter is about. What follows is a range of perspectives on common worries and fears. The voices presented are ones you would likely hear in a support group. Most of the quotes are taken directly from notes made by myself and my colleague, Dr. Claire Edmonds, on the therapy groups we led together for a research study at the Healing Journey Program at Princess Margaret Hospital and from homework assignments done by the participants. Hopefully reading these quotes will be like bringing a support group into the privacy of your own home. The advantage of a support group is the wealth of experiences and perspectives brought forward by the many voices; voices that reflect good days and bad days, voices that inspire and challenge us to live fully and meaningfully and voices that capture those times when nothing seems to be going well and the outlook and one's capacity to face it, looms as bleak and hopeless.

At whatever point you find yourself, there is always the opportunity to be heard and supported. No matter where you are on your journey or what you are feeling, there is always hope. Hope can mean different things at different times; but at its most basic, hope means the possibility of lightening your load and opening your heart and spirit to a wider perspective than the one presently holding you in its grip.

The following describes some of the more common worries that come up time and time again in support groups. Perhaps you will see your own worries reflected here. If so, you are already on a healing path. Finding our words in the words of others helps us to feel supported and understood. Knowing others have felt the way you do may give you the impetus to start your own healing path. Even if you don't find your worries and fears described here, perhaps reading the concerns of others will help you to understand how you are different, and in doing so begin a process that will ultimately take you in your own healing direction.

First, I will present the voices that reflect turmoil on a number of different issues. In each case, after the chorus of troubled voices, I will present other perspectives. These are the voices of patients who have worked through some of the turmoil and found more peaceful resolutions. Still, the apparent leap from the troubled voice to a more peaceful perspective is deceptive. At first glance, it seems as if someone has waved a magic wand transforming instantly the worried thought into a more calming affirmation. I wish there were such a magic wand. But achieving a more peaceful frame of mind requires some determination and practice on your part. It is not enough to read about it. Often the feelings of sadness, anger or hurt associated with the troubled thoughts need time to be acknowledged and felt before it is even possible to consider another perspective. The good news is it can be done. Greater peace of mind is achievable.

This book is about supporting you through that process with the aid of these voices of experience. First we will document them. Then we will do the challenging work of learning to manage our thoughts more effectively. This chapter describes them, the next chapter takes you through the step-by-step process of noticing and reframing your worries and fears.

Guilt and Blame

When people are first diagnosed with cancer, they often dwell on all the things that could have been done differently and blame themselves or others for the current situation. These thoughts orbit obsessively around a list of "shoulds" and "should nots."

I should have gone to the doctor earlier.

I shouldn't have stayed in that stressful situation at work. I knew it wasn't good for me.

Maybe I should have exercised more or become a vegetarian.

I should have ended that negative relationship earlier.

I blame my doctor. She told me there was nothing to worry about. I also blame myself. I shouldn't have trusted her.

Guilt isn't limited to past behavior. It can flourish in thoughts about the future and worries about becoming a burden to family, friends or work associates. This focus on being a burden is very common. It is particularly difficult for those who have always taken on the care of others. For example, middle aged women who have cared for aging parents and children whether they be toddlers, teenagers or young adults do not find it easy to be in the position of needing to look after themselves. The idea is foreign to them. Life is already so much of a balancing act. The thought of taking time for themselves for treatment and care makes them feel selfish! How will they continue to do all the things they have been used to doing for others if they have to go through surgery, chemo and radiation. Worse, they cannot imagine depending on others for care. People who give help freely often find it hard to ask for help.

Similar thoughts plague those who have been totally self-reliant and independent. Suddenly they are in the position of possibly needing to rely on others and the very thought is unacceptable. Perhaps they will need assistance with executing an important work project or require help for instrumental tasks, like transport to and from the hospital, or cutting the lawn, or cooking meals. They too find it very difficult to ask for help and dwell on this idea that they will become burdensome to others.

One of the most gut wrenching issues, frequently expressed in support groups by cancer patients, is the belief that now their children are much more susceptible to cancer. This idea can eat away at them. In cases where genetic testing is possible, the anxiety is often played out in intense soul searching. Is it better to know or not to know and what are the ramifications of each position? Finding peace of mind through this process can be a challenge.

If all this were not enough guilt for cancer patients to encounter and manage, worries about being well enough to participate in important social or professional activities play on their minds. For example, cancer patients often express feelings of guilt, more so than disappointment, when they need to rest instead of joining in family activities or excursions or cannot make future plans for outings or travel because they don't know whether they will be well enough to participate. Many parents and partners express feelings of guilt that their children or spouses are saddled with the experience of having an ill parent or partner rather than having a "normal" one. They feel responsible for this outcome.

I know it doesn't make sense, but I feel like I'm letting my family down.

I'm worried that now my daughter will get breast cancer too and it is my fault.

Does this mean my son will get prostate cancer?

What if I become a burden to my family and friends?

I feel sad that my husband now has to live with pain and fear of loss and I can't make it go away.

Will I become helpless as the illness progresses? Will I become a burden to my family?

In a support group when these kinds of feelings are expressed, they are immediately understood because everyone can relate in an immediate and visceral way. Their common experience helps them to understand these points of view in ways friends or family members may not. At any given time in a group, there is likely to be someone struggling with the same thing or has a past experience of similar thoughts and feelings. Often people share their own perspectives of these experiences and these different viewpoints can help shift feelings of guilt and blame to more peaceful thoughts and feelings. Here are some examples:

Cancer is a complex process. I don't know what caused my cancer. It could be any combination of many factors. It doesn't make any sense to blame myself for my cancer. I have it. What am I going to do about it? That's the important question. How am I going to use what I'm learning here to help myself get better?

What's past is past. I don't have to go down that negative spiral of blaming myself or others.

What's most important now is my healing and how I can help myself move forward.

I don't know whether my daughter will get breast cancer or not. No one can know that for sure. But I do know my daughter has a lot of love in her life and lots of resources. I now have a chance to model for her some things that may help her later in life like expressing emotions more openly and finding ways of dealing with fear.

My husband and I can talk about fears and sorrows. We are trying to live in the present with each other as much as possible. He has an inner strength and goodness that will help him get through this.

"There's a change in my attitude. I don't feel like I'm burdening others so much anymore. It helped me to see it from my friend's point of view. She said "If the tables were turned and you were helping me, would you think I was being a burden to you?" Of course, I wouldn't. So when I start to feel guilty, I think about what she said and it helps.

I grew up in a family that didn't have health. Both my parents were unwell at times. I never felt we didn't have a good life.

I couldn't go to the family party on Sunday. Instead of feeling guilty, or getting mad at myself, I said, "This is fine.

This is what my body needs. I'm not giving in to the illness. I'm looking after myself."

I don't know what is ahead and there is no point worrying about the unknown. My family will love me no matter how I will be.

I was angry and disappointed with myself. Now, I'm gentler. I don't get mad at myself. I'm working on having better mental thoughts.

Why Me?

This Shouldn't Be Happening to Me Because

- I'm too young.
- My children need me.
- I've worked hard all my life and I haven't had a chance to enjoy retirement.
- I have always been healthy. I exercised regularly, never smoked and was always careful about what I ate.
- I don't deserve this. I'm a good person.

Unwelcome and unexpected, cancer also seems unfair at times. For some, there is considerable turmoil around the thought: "This shouldn't be happening to me." In the case of children or young parents, cancer seems particularly unfair. The quiet pall that settles over a support group, when a young mother describes her disbelief and despair about having cancer and the thought of leaving her children, is palpable. The turmoil is also strong in people who have made a point of looking after themselves and their health or who have worked hard or lived virtuously and expected rewards for such dedication. In addition, the daily schedule that used to revolve around work, family and relationships now has to accommodate cancer, with its many doctor and hospital visits, tests and procedures and demands on time, money and wellbeing. The experience of the hospital itself is often unpleasant with its cacophony of sights, sounds and smells. Resentment naturally builds and peace of mind deteriorates.

Why did I have to get this where there are so many terrible people in the world that are perfectly healthy?

I'm being cheated of all the plans my wife and I have made for the future. I feel I'm putting in all the time to build and maintain a strong relationship, but it will be someone else that will share those moments without earning the rights to them.

I don't belong here. I have small children at home who need me. No one knows or loves them the way I do. How can I have cancer? How can I look them in the eyes and even think of being anywhere else? I can't leave them. I need to be around. I need to beat this thing. The doctors don't give me much hope.

Sometimes, there are no immediate words of comfort. Take for example, the young mother, quoted above, who fears leaving her children. If there is any comfort at all in these moments, it is more about having her raw pain acknowledged than anything else. And that indeed is something. In the support group, she is heard in an attentive, caring, way. For a moment her pain is held and shared and that process may begin to shift the weight of suffering. In such a situation, I might say, "I hear how difficult this is for you. I also hear your determination to be around for your children. We are here to listen and we care about what is happening to you. Right now you're feeling angry and vulnerable and hope seems a long way off. I expect most people here can relate to moments like that." Then, I would turn to the group as a whole and ask "What does hope mean to you? How do you find hope?"

Many stories and perspectives about hope and living fully emerge in response to these questions. We will be continually exploring this throughout the book, as hope is an important nutrient in calming the mind and warming the heart. When more peaceful ways of looking at the situation do not come to mind, there are still many ways of warming the heart. For now, here are some other perspectives on the "Why me?" question.

I never had this "Why me?" feeling. Why not me? Where is it written that there are any guarantees of a healthy long life? We can't control the cards that are dealt to us; we can only play the hand that we are dealt to the best of our ability.

I was angry at first. It seemed so unfair. But I'm trying to get beyond fear and anger. I'm trying to be more atune to how my body is reacting and to stand outside myself and be the observer. When I'm angry, my body is tense and charged, and my thoughts are racing. I'm learning my anger doesn't help me. I'm learning not to react so much.

When I think of leaving my children, my heart and mind go haywire. I tell myself, "I'm here now. No one knows what will happen in the future. Concentrate on now. Now is all we ever have."

I'm wasting precious time and energy getting worked up about this. I find The Serenity Prayer really helps: "God grant me the serenity to accept the things I cannot change; courage to change the things I can; and wisdom to know the difference."

Losses: Hair, Attractiveness, Health, Work, Mobility . . . Identity

Cancer can surprise us with some unexpected challenges. People expect to face whatever difficulties are associated with treatment, but they may be taken aback by psychological or existential questions that arise from losses associated with the illness. Who am I if I'm not working? Who am I if I'm not contributing to society? Who am I if I am not looking attractive or radiating health? Who am I if I can't look after my children? Who am I if I can't do the things I'm used to doing?

Take the case of Barbara. She had always been proud of her natural blonde hair. She considered it her most attractive asset. So when she looked in the mirror and saw a bald head, her mind went AHHH with shock. The dramatic change in her appearance was symbolic of all the other changes she has had to undergo because of cancer: how her life has slowed down and become controlled by doctors appointments; how she depended on others for occasional help when she used to do everything herself; how she was unsure about who she is without her job and yet unsure whether she wanted to go back; how she could no longer go for long hikes because she is always so tired. Still, as she recounted all this to the group, she laughed at herself. "All those years, I fussed about my hair. For what?"

Another group member agreed, "When I looked into the mirror, I have a feeling of fading. My hair is falling out, my eyebrows are falling out and I think, 'I'm fading out of the picture. I'm fading out of my life.'"

Here are some more comments along a similar vein:

I hate looking in the mirror. It's not me. I don't like my image. I smile through it a lot . . . putting on a brave face.

What a thief cancer is.

At moments I feel so totally helpless, ill and discouraged. The helpless feeling comes from the fact I'm not able to do the things I used to be able to do – most importantly, looking after my children. My body functions differently. I have no energy; I'm nauseous; I can't eat. There's a sense of total weakness. With all this comes a feeling of bleakness and total discouragement.

If you don't have health, you don't have anything.

I used to see myself as a strong person. I could do anything. Now, I see myself as weak. I feel useless because I can't do the things I used to. I think these feelings of uselessness come from the protestant work ethic my parents instilled in me. You're only a good person if you work.

I'm not a productive member of society. I'm not doing anything. My body is betraying me.

These thoughts erode confidence and undermine self worth. It is hard enough to go through the experience of illness without adding the burden of loss of self esteem. And of course there are good days and bad days: on the good ones, there is a feeling of empowerment – of being able to take these challenges in stride. On the bad days, these thoughts can be overwhelming, leaving a person feeling dejected and unworthy. Here are some more peaceful perspectives from others who have had similar thoughts.

Cancer may alter my physical appearance but I can't let it touch the core of who I am.

People, who matter deeply, care about you regardless of how you look. That is what kept me going.

When I stepped out of the bath and looked in the mirror, I saw this skinny ravaged body. I hate what I see. I feel like my life has been ravaged. But then I try to put these feelings into perspective. I tell myself, "You're here. That's what counts. Celebrate that."

I've told others, this is the way I am. I'm bald. Accept me.

I'm not going to let illness or my job define who I am. My self-worth comes from knowing what is most meaningful and important to me and living my life in a way that reflects that.

I dispute the idea that "If you don't have health, you don't have anything." I'm working really hard at not making that true. I think it's about being . . . not doing. I can't do the things I used to, but that doesn't mean I don't have anything. I've learned to really enjoy and relish moments of just being. For example, when my son comes in to say goodnight to me each night and reaches for my hand, watching my daughter cook in the kitchen with me helping from the chair. There's a lot of living in those moments.

I'm coming to see that cancer has been positive in many ways: living more in the present, being happier with what I do have, living with deeper values. I was more depressed when I was well and had a lot of things going for me. Now, I rarely feel that way. Now I have so much to live for.

Waiting

The cancer journey is often about Waiting. Waiting to hear back from the doctor; waiting for a referral; waiting for treatment to begin; waiting for test results; waiting long past scheduled time for appointments in the hospital, waiting for the post treatment check up. In waiting time, the mind can be particularly restless and inventive. It seems to take perverse delight in conjuring the worst case scenario. There are two important things to remember. First, waiting is hard. Nearly everyone acknowledges it. The worry and restlessness associated with waiting brings a chorus of recognition and empathy in support groups. So be gentle with yourself at these times. Second, whatever you can do to let go of some of this anticipatory worry will help you in the long run, since waiting is an intrinsic part of the cancer experience and presents itself in many facets. Learning to manage the fears and restlessness associated with waiting is a key ingredient in regaining some control over your response to your illness. You don't need to be a passive recipient. What eventually happens may be outside of your control, but how you respond is up to you. The next chapter will present many ideas for discharging restless energy. Here are some experiences and perspectives on waiting.

It's the waiting that's hard.

It's the not-knowing that I find so hard to deal with – waiting to find out.

I find myself very caught up in the whole thing when something's going on and I'm waiting to hear. I can't get it out of my mind. I'm fretting: going over and over the same thing.

I'm waiting for treatment to start and I keep imagining things going wrong.

Although waiting is hard, some people do manage the restlessness and worry that comes with it, at least some of the time:

Two years ago, when I was waiting for news, I was panicking inside. Now, I'm fine tuning things. So waiting is a different kind of waiting. Whatever the results are, they are. How I respond is my attitude.

I'm anxious because I'm waiting to hear the result of my scans. I notice when I take time to read spiritual or healing material the anxiety goes away. I'm going to take time to do this today and during the week.

I used to spend so much time worrying about what might happen. You can spend a lot of time worrying about test results. Why waste time doing that? You'll deal with it when the time comes. A lot of times, I stop myself from going overboard.

I used to get so upset when I had to wait so long for my appointments. Now I come prepared to wait. I tell myself, it will take whatever time it will take and I'm not going to get upset. I bring books and my knitting and I find it very meditative to sit quietly and knit.

I have to wait for the biopsy results. But I believe that I can live completely with sorrow and joy, holding all my very precious reactions to this disease and the unknown nature of this journey.

Doctors

A good relationship with one's doctor and health care team is a critical component of peace of mind for the patient. A patient needs to feel comfortable asking questions, expressing concerns and to be fully informed about treatment options. In my experience, most patients are satisfied and grateful for the care they are receiving. They know and appreciate that their doctors are hard working, well-intended and dealing with complex and demanding workloads.

However some doctors can undermine patients' wellbeing by being dismissive, inattentive, unavailable or perfunctory – not allowing time for comments or questions. If such a pattern persists, the patient may be better off switching to another physician. Support groups are helpful in encouraging fellow members not to accept conditions in which this kind of trust, support and care are lacking. They urge fellow members to seek out physicians who will listen respectfully and appropriately to concerns and to get second opinions if they are uncertain or uneasy about treatment protocols. Helpful suggestions are also exchanged such as making a list of questions and concerns before meeting with the doctor and taking a partner or companion who can take notes.

The way doctors communicate with patients has a profound effect on their wellbeing. In recent years, more emphasis has been placed in medical training on how to communicate difficult news to patients and their families. This is a welcome development. Over the years, I have heard many stories from patients and family members about the insensitive manner in which bad news was delivered to them. One woman was told, "The wolf is nipping at your heels and the wolf is going to get you." Another woman was told she "might as well order the pine box." These are extreme examples. Most often the stories reflect a more common and thoughtless lack of care: such as being told the news in passing from a doorway, or while one is naked and vulnerable on the examining table, or without any apparent recognition of what it is like to receive such news. This lack of basic human connection at such a time has an unsettling and disheartening effect which can persist in the minds and hearts of patients and their loved ones.

It is important to re-iterate that most patients enjoy a good relationship with their doctors. I don't want to paint a picture of insensitive and uncaring doctors. Nothing could be further from the truth. But in those cases where things go wrong in the doctor patient relationship, they often go very wrong, stirring significant unrest and upheaval in the mind. Sometimes patients are literally haunted by the words of their physicians. Such was the case with Alison.

Alison went into her doctor's office feeling physically well and confident about all the extra things she was doing to take care of herself. She had joined the Healing Journey Program, had started a program of exercise, was eating well and was seeing a naturopath. She left her doctor's office feeling "shattered." She reported being a "wreck for days," retreating into solitude, crying frequently, eating poorly, and feeling without hope. Nothing had changed in the physical status of her disease. In fact, the news was good since the latest scans showed some shrinkage in the size of the tumors in her liver and overall her condition was considered stable. But the words of her doctor haunted her. He warned her this period of stability would not last since the "cancer wants to grow" and he reminded her that her condition was "terminal." Even a month later, the blunt words of her oncologist "are always with me, like a shadow."

Alison was fortunate to be part of a support group in which wise voices could help her see that one doctor's careless choice of words needn't take away her hope. She was the best judge of how she was feeling and if she believed the extra things she was doing were helpful to her, who was to say they were not? They also worked at exorcising the power of the physicians specific words "the cancer wants to grow" by telling their own perspectives and helping Alison to reframe the words and their meaning so they did not exert such power over her.

Significant turmoil also results in cases where patients and family members believe doctors have been negligent resulting in a delay in diagnosis or a misdiagnosis. What if these mistakes cost the patient his or her life? The mind reels with anger, betrayal, and sadness. Trust in the medical system is likely shattered. Naturally it takes some time to work through these feelings before any peace of mind is possible. A first step is recognizing the toll such feelings take on your wellbeing. We will discuss this more in the section on forgiveness in chapter five, Warming the Troubled Heart. Many people find journaling helps in this situation: getting all your angry and hurt feelings down on paper. Remember, this is a process. It takes time to shift away from these feelings toward a calmer mind. Part of the process is recognizing this and allowing time for acknowledging and expressing your authentic feelings around the issue.

I am angry with those doctors who misdiagnosed me. Perhaps the delay will cost me my life. I get angrier and angrier every time I think about it. It eats away at me.

The doctor was blunt with me. I was completely devastated by her words. I can't get them out of my mind.

My doctor always seems to be in a hurry. Before I can get to my list, he's out the door.

Without this group, I don't know where I'd be. They encouraged me to get a second opinion and it has made all the difference.

I wouldn't have done it without their support. Now, I'm doing well with this new treatment.

I have complete trust in my doctor. She really listens and cares about her patients. I have the sense that whatever happens, she will be there for me. She won't abandon me.

My doctor asked me with seeming interest if there was anything we had missed on my list. I loved that doctor.

It was bad news, but the doctor was very kind. Before I left the office, he asked me, "What's most on your mind?" I was really touched by that question.

Worries About Treatment Starting; Worries About Treatment Ending

People often find treatment is not as bad as they anticipated. Sometimes, people join support groups after diagnosis, but before treatment begins and they usually leave their first session feeling much relieved. They've learned from the descriptions of others that treatment is not likely to be as difficult as they fear. The hard part, they're told, is the waiting. That is when worrying is at its peak. Of course, people react differently to the same treatment and there are a wide variety of treatment protocols and procedures. Many do have a tough time of it. No one can predict with complete accuracy what it is going to be like for anyone else. Nonetheless, once treatment starts, worrying generally subsides. The experience is no longer an unknown commodity and focus naturally changes from worried anticipation to getting through whatever challenges treatment brings.

Not only do people worry about beginning treatment, they also worry about treatment ending. It is not as paradoxical as it sounds. Of course there is the relief of not having to endure more chemo or radiation, but there is also the worry about ending these powerful forces whose sole design is to eradicate cancer cells. While actively engaged in treatment, there is the comfortable sense that everything is being done to fight the cancer. Once that stops, there is often anxiety around "What now?" and the uneasy prospect of less engagement with the medical system that many see as their sole ongoing protector and insurance against their disease. Often personal relationships have been forged with the health care team and the ending of treatment brings a sense of loss of care, security, and the fellowship that was fostered around the regular schedule of attention and care.

Family and friends tend to see the end of treatment as the end of the illness and expect that now the patient can return to their normal life. The patient is often both physically and emotionally exhausted and does not always share this sentiment. So what others expect will be a time of joy and celebration may well be a time of anxiety and exhaustion for the patient.

Here are some of the worries expressed about treatment, procedures and the end of treatment:

I was very anxious about the procedures of drawing blood and getting hooked up to chemo as well as the after-effects.

I'm worried the chemo will make me really sick and I won't enjoy my time with my daughter who is visiting for a short time.

I'm worried about having a porta-cath inserted. I've been poked and prodded enough. I'm afraid of pain.

I'm worried about having anticipatory nausea like I did last time.

I'm worried I will have more trouble recovering from this treatment as I don't feel very well already and I'm concerned this will affect my vacation with my family.

I found the daily visits to the hospital quite depressing — -seeing so many patients in terribly wasted and debilitating conditions and anticipating my own future.

I expected to be so relieved when treatment ended, but I wasn't. My family and friends celebrated with a big cake. I put on a good face, but inside, I felt numb.

Looking back, I think the end of treatment was one of the hardest times. My family acted as if now the worries were behind us. The cancer is gone. End of story. But it didn't feel like the end to me. While I was in treatment, there was always something to do. I didn't have to think. It was about getting through it. But once the treatment was over, it was like all the emotion caught up with me and I felt it wash over me, swamp-ing me like a wave.

Here are some more peaceful perspectives on the same issues:

The porta-cath means that I will only need one injection. I will be able to handle the brief moment of discomfort and then I won't have to deal with any more pain.

I'm learning to quiet my mind and put my fears in perspective.

My body has handled chemo very well. During most of the past six months, I have felt energetic and well. The tiredness and run down feeling I'm experiencing now is typical of chemo treatment and less severe than many experience. I can still continue doing most things I like to do, but I just need to rest more often and slow down.

When I think chemo, I'm not thinking poison. I'm thinking healing. I'm determined to have a good experience.

I spoke with the doctor and nurse about the needle biopsy before we started. They both said their patients usually did not complain about pain. They showed me the tiny needles they used. They said if I felt pain to say so and they would stop the procedure. We discussed the anxiety related to a procedure like this. They were both aware that this was a fairly emotional and anxious time for my husband and me. I think all these things helped to make the biopsy more comfortable. There was a gentle feeling in the room.

The end of treatment was unsettling for me. What happens if it didn't work? What happens if the cancer comes back? My next check-up seemed a long time away. That is when I got interested in my own healing resources. I now have a regular daily practice of relaxation, meditation and journaling. It not only makes me feel better, but it helps me believe I'm doing everything I possibly can to stay well.

New Symptoms: Worries About Recurrence

One remark that gets everyone nodding in a support group because it is so universally experienced is the comment, "Whenever I get a new symptom, I think the cancer is on the move. If I have a headache, I worry it's a brain tumor. If I have a backache, I think, "Now it's in my spine. Why do I do this to myself? I go through all this agony and it turns out to be nothing."

Most often, a headache is simply that: a headache, not a brain tumor. However, a suggestion that has worked for many is to make a pact with yourself not to worry for a period of time, perhaps three days, perhaps ten days, whatever seems appropriate. During that time, keep a log of your symptoms. When you start to worry, remind yourself of your pact, "I'm not going to worry for this period of three (or whatever number you have chosen) days. Instead I'm keeping a log. If after the specified days, I'm still concerned, I will seek out appropriate medical attention and I will have a detailed list of my symptoms to help the investigation of what this might be."

Being a member of a support group helps because you learn heightened sensitivity to new symptoms is simply part of the experience of having cancer. You hear many stories of people who had similar worries and their symptoms either went away or turned out to be something other than cancer. They worried needlessly. But what if your worries are well founded? What if the new symptoms do point to active disease? Again, being in a support group helps because there will likely be people in the group who have had a recurrence and can reassure you that it is not the end of the world. There are still treatment options available to them and they find ways of living fully and meaningfully with this new stage in their journey. More often than not, their example will give you hope.

My back really aches. Could it be cancer in the bone? When I have a headache, I worry about having a brain tumor.

The moment I feel physical pain, I'm down in the dumps.

I woke up yesterday with a sore shoulder, neck and chest and I immediately thought the cancer is on the move. I also felt an enlarged node in my neck. I try to tell myself, I often have this ache in my neck and shoulder from a neck injury and that I really am OK. I think about having long living genes in my family and that I will live long. Today, the ache in my neck is better, maybe the cancer is not on the move. I can still feel the enlarged lymph node. This causes fear so I try to meditate and make myself quiet. This helps and I went out to a party and felt much better.

I don't have to do this to myself. I know this new pain in my shoulders is probably from all the gardening I did yesterday. It doesn't help me to get so worked up. I need to stay calm and enjoy my day.

I've had this back ache for years. Chemo may have added to the aches. Yoga may help me.

I received my CEA results last week, only to find the levels elevated 50 percent, which indicates the cancer has developed a resistance to the chemo we are currently using. My immediate response was that "cold" feeling running through

*my entire body. However within a matter of a couple of min-
utes I was totally calm and relaxed and ready to investigate
the next step of the medical process. I was able to leave
behind the fear and sense of being discouraged and replace it
with calmness. I was able to draw on my meditation practice
and call on the calm I receive from it. I thought to myself, this
is just a minor setback in the tour to wellness. Many others
have gone through the same thing.*

Uncertain Future

This is the big one: the central fear we talked about earlier
in the chapter. We look for reassurance that everything will be
fine. We want someone to tell us with 100 percent certainty that
we need only submit ourselves to the recommended treatment
and we will be cured. The cancer will be gone. It will never come
back and we will live in good health until a ripe old age.
Unfortunately, no one can give you this guarantee and the
absence of it creates distress. Naturally, you yearn for this outcome. Gradually the realization dawns that there never have
been any guarantees of good health or a long life for you or anyone else, but such realization doesn't always help us deal with
the anxiety. This, like so many other new perspectives, takes
time.

Our uncertain future is often with us and can undermine our
enjoyment of life if we allow it to take over our minds. Holidays
and celebrations naturally carry a tinge of sadness and longing
as you wonder whether you will be present the following year.
Bigger questions and feelings arise when you contemplate the
possibility of not being around for the people you love. Even if
you repress immediately any thought of dying, these thoughts
can creep up on you in the middle of the night or watching a
movie or at some other unexpected moment.

Sometimes it is not our own mortality that is most on our
minds, but our capabilities to live fully and meaningfully if more
treatment is required or if our symptoms get worse and don't
respond to treatment. As one man put it, "I don't want to live a
half-life. I'd rather be dead." Sometimes we wonder if we will
have the courage to go on if things get worse.

Since we don't know for sure what lies ahead, it is often difficult to plan trips or family outings several months away.
Sometimes even planning the next day is problematic; you don't

know if you are going to feel well enough for the activity planned and perhaps you begin to feel annoyed, despondent, or trapped by these circumstances. Whatever the case, living with uncertainty is difficult:

I don't want the unknown to hit me with a big boot.

I can't bear the thought that I might not be there for my children's graduations, weddings, and the births of grandchildren.

I went to church for the evening Christmas Carol Service and during the service, I wondered if I will be here for this service next year. During the songs, I felt all teary and during the final solo I almost started to cry thinking I would like that sung at my funeral.

I have sad thoughts when I hear Christmas music, wondering if this will be my last Christmas. How will my daughter and husband cope if I die? And what about the rest of my family?

I wonder how I can have a strong will to live and yet also die in peace if I can't control the progression of this cancer. Sometimes I wonder if I'm preparing for living or for dying and what the difference is.

I'm worried I will get frightened or discouraged and give up.

I wonder how well I will cope if the symptoms get worse or if I need more intrusive treatments.

Facing our fears is the first step. Not backing away from them. This does not mean we have to live constantly with our fears. Sometimes pushing them away is an effective strategy for a while. But ultimately, if we are to have any lasting peace of mind, acknowledging our fears is the first step. This awareness brings new opportunities to work with the fear and to reframe it for oneself in a way that "feels right." It is ultimately a chance to find new meaning or perspective and to re-engage fully and meaningfully in life. Essentially this is what this entire book is about. For the moment, here are some examples of how others reframed their fears, found new meaning and sought to re-engage in life fully when faced with thoughts of the uncertain future we all share:

Reframing

We all have a death sentence. It's part of being alive.

When nothing is sure, anything is possible.

I've decided to live my life as if I have a future.

As long as I'm alive, there is always a chance of getting better, not only of getting worse. I need to remember that.

When I experience fear, I say to myself: "This is just a thought. I'm having one of those fear thoughts. It's not going to last forever. I'm not going to let myself be pulled down by it."

Making Sense of It All

I think I can gradually become more able to "surrender" to whatever happens with strength and a belief in divine guidance. I realize this is a process that takes time. I have a big psychological adjustment to make to accept the uncertainty of my future.

I'm not religious but I am spiritual. I don't need to understand everything. I accept there are some things beyond my understanding. I'm okay with that. I don't know whether my illness was pre-ordained. I don't care. Maybe, maybe not. It doesn't really matter. The important thing I've learned to accept what is. Then I can move to "What can I do now? From a stronger perspective."

Living Fully

I think it is important to live with reverence. Live because you want to live not because you fear death. It was an important thing for me to learn.

I don't focus on the future. It is enough to have one good day. One good day may lead to another good day. My whole life is this one day. The past doesn't exist. The future – who knows? If I'm able to live one good day, I can be content.

When and how I die is beyond my control. But we have resources to manage our fears. We can control how we respond to the things that weigh heavily on us. I don't want a fear of death to control the way I live my life. I want to live my life from a place of strength, not a place of fear. I have a strong will to live."

Despair: "I Can't Take This Anymore"

I had a very good friend who lived many years with breast cancer. Most of those years were good ones, but I remember once when I asked her how she was doing, she replied "Just shoot me." She had had enough. What bothered her most was for too long a period she felt she had had no break from the disease. Just as she was starting to feel better, something else would happen and she was back in "cancerland." How she longed for a normal morning, when she might wake up free of worry and pain, make a cup of coffee and read the paper. Was that too much to ask? That's all she wanted, a morning without cancer. She felt so weary of the whole process and the unrelenting way it took over her life.

Periods of sadness and despair are normal. They only become a problem when you stay stuck in them. Then you need help. A good place to start is your family physician. Often the hospital where you receive or received treatment has support programs and trained health professionals who can also give you guidance at such times. It is important to get help when a period of despondency settles in for more than a few days at a time.

However, having a down day, or even several down days is okay. I use the word "okay" because so many people believe it is not okay to have negative thoughts. There is a popular notion that "thinking positively" is an essential part of healing and if you entertain any negative thought, you are doing yourself and your illness a disservice. This is an unfair burden and responsibility to place upon yourself or let others place upon you. While common sense and our own experience tell us we feel better when we think positively and worse when we think negatively, this does not mean it is unhealthy to have a negative thought or period of downheartedness. As we have already discussed, allowing authentic feelings to come forward is an important part of healing. Sometimes it comes as a relief to drop the "brave face" one has put on for the world, or for oneself, and let more "negative," but authentic feelings come to the surface. In my experience, most everyone can identify with the group member who describes feeling upset and despondent about things and then adds with fervor "If one more person tells me to "just think positively, I'm going to scream!" Allow yourself to have your feelings without shutting them down.

Sometimes going through treatment is so tiring that even setting one foot out of bed requires tremendous effort and again, it's okay to have a day like that where everything seems to require too much and feelings of dismay and hopelessness set in. Sometimes the need arises to speak more frankly about what the situation is like for you and when you find that no one else wants to hear or they simply can't or won't understand what it's like for you, feelings of alienation and loneliness can settle in for a while.

Again, we'll be talking more about this in the section on finding warmth, meaning and spirit, but right now what is important to know is it is perfectly normal to have days like this. Take heart from the likelihood these feelings will pass.

What's the point? . . . What's the point? . . . What's the point?

I've been in a ball weeping for days. I ask myself, "Is the struggle worth it? "

It feels like waiting. It doesn't feel like living.

I feel marginalized. Isolated. Alone.

I feel more depressed, less optimistic than usual and I'm afraid this will slow down my healing.

Accepting that feelings of sadness and despair are part of the journey and that most likely they will come and go may give you some reassurance and solace on such days. Here are some wise voices on the subject:

Although I find fear very uncomfortable to live with at times, I know somehow that this feeling will pass, like all mental/emotional states and I can imagine things getting better during those times.

Feeling depressed at times is something I have had to accept like most people with cancer. I will take the rest of the morning to do things to try to help with this. I will meditate, listen to relaxation tape, and notice my reactions.

Feeling down is not going to affect my immune system, but holding in the sadness and disappointment will. I am working on releasing these feelings in some way each day.

Feelings of sadness are normal in my situation. They will come and go. I don't seem to get "stuck" inside them for too long. One thing I do to try to help with this is to think about all the things I'm grateful for before I go to sleep. There are always lots.

I have learned there are good times and bad times in this cancer journey. I can learn to live through them.

There are rhythms and sometimes the rhythms are down. You just live through it.

Am I Doing Enough to Fight my Cancer?

As if you don't have enough on your mind, another worry that often plagues cancer patients and their loved ones is the question of whether enough is being done to fight the cancer. Well meaning friends and family members are forever coming up with new cures they have heard about and may press you to try them. Often there may be little or no substance for their claims. The internet is both a helpful and confusing source of information. How do you sort out what is potentially helpful from what is potentially harmful or useless in your case? The array of alternative therapies can present like a baffling cornucopia of possibilities and quackery. Perhaps your rational mind leads you in one direction and your emotions in another. You certainly can't try them all. How do you choose what response to all this information is best for you? What if you miss that one idea or therapy that could make a difference? The thought is crazy making.

There are so many possible cures and unconventional treatments. Am I doing the right things? Maybe there are some things that might help me more? How do I decide what to choose?

I get so irritated by all the people who force their own ideas on me about what is best for my health. One moment it is shark cartiledge, the next it is a blueberry extract or a new tea.

I wish somebody could tell me, this is what you need to do in a convincing way. It is all so confusing.

In support groups, participants describe their own exploration of conventional and alternative approaches and how they handle the unsolicited comments and advice from others. The range of stories is often helpful as people learn there are different needs for more or less information at different points in the journey of cancer diagnosis and treatment. Everyone can identify with the struggle of finding one's own level of comfort with the degree to which they seek out new information and remedies and the point at which they declare, "I'm happy with the decisions I've made and what I'm doing to fight my cancer. I don't need the aggravation and confusion of more information or advice right now."

Support group leaders often need to rein in discussions that would otherwise veer into lengthy accounts of a particular approach and bring the group back to focus on the common underlying issues and fears. As so often is the case, the central underlying anxiety relates to the difficulty of living with uncertainty and the fact there is no certain answer to the question, "What do I need to do to eradicate my cancer and ensure it never comes back?"

If there were a single therapy, conventional or alternative, that effectively eradicated all cancer, we would know about it. So the challenge is to find a level of trust with the choices you have made and to take comfort from the knowledge this is all you can do. Many find sustenance in their inner journeys as a complement to their conventional treatment: using mind, body and spirit to promote healing. This book will assist you along that pathway.

I can't do everything. I feel the things I have been doing are right for me so I might as well trust my inner wisdom instead of getting anxious about it.

What I like about the inner work I'm doing – meditation, relaxation and imagery – is that it gives me the sense I'm doing everything I can to fight the cancer by creating optimal conditions for healing to take place. If my body, mind and spirit are relaxed and peaceful, my body is in a much better position to fight the cancer than if my body, mind and spirit are anxious and stressed. I really believe that.

Documenting the troubled mind is a first step toward healing. Whether this is a good day or a bad day, there is always the possibility of an opening: of moving away from feelings of distress toward feelings of greater comfort and ease. Hopefully it is comforting to know that you are not alone with your troubled thoughts and perhaps you have been helped or inspired by the range of voices dealing with similar issues. But the crux of the matter remains: How can you manage your own thoughts more effectively and experience greater peace of mind? The next two chapters will help you: chapter two presents strategies for managing your thoughts and chapter three teaches basic skills to calm your body and mind. A wide range of experienced voices will guide you.

Two
Calming Your Mind

How do you stop the thoughts?
That's what I want to know.

Thoughts create our experience. For example, how much of your suffering is directly attributed to cancer and how much to your thoughts about cancer? Yes, there are times when the disease itself brings discomfort and pain but even then, part of your suffering is likely related to the meaning you attribute to the new pain or suffering rather than the illness itself.

The fact is our thoughts create much of our suffering. So how do you stop the thoughts? I wish I knew. I have never met anyone who can. But it is possible to manage your thoughts more effectively. You can learn to respond to your thoughts in new ways. It takes some effort and persistence, but the good news is it can be done. You can gradually learn to direct your thoughts away from distress toward greater peace of mind.

The crux of the matter is this: you might not be able to control the course of your cancer, but you can control how you respond to it. This is a very liberating idea. You need not be a passive recipient of your distressing thoughts. You can choose to respond in ways that diminish your suffering and increase your wellbeing.

You Are What You Think:

We've all heard the expression "You are what you eat." Well, it may be more accurate to say "You are what you think." Our daily diet of thoughts has as much effect on our wellbeing as our daily diet of food. What we put into our minds is every bit as important, perhaps more so, than what we put into our bodies.

When you consider how much attention our culture places on the quality of food and diet on the appearance and health of the human body, it is disappointing that so little concern is given to the quality of thoughts on our overall health. The link is just as direct: by making wise choices with the food we eat, we can produce healthier bodies; by making wise choices with the thoughts we think, we can produce healthier minds, bodies and spirits.

"So what?" you might say. "I can control the food I put into my body but I can't stop the thoughts from coming into my head." True, you would have to be a saint or superman to have complete control over your thoughts. But you can learn to work with them and to respond in new ways. With time and repeated practice, these strategies can bring greater health and happiness. They can bring you a calm mind and a warm heart.

The potential impact on wellbeing is so great it really is a mystery why more attention has not been directed to these simple strategies. They could be taught in elementary school alongside good nutritional habits. No doubt the time will come when such instruction is mainstream. But in the meantime, let's start with basics – recognizing the impact of your thoughts on your wellbeing.

Noticing How Your Thoughts Affect Your Wellbeing

What happens when you are in the grip of repetitive and disturbing thoughts about your illness? Managing thoughts more effectively begins with noticing. Indeed noticing is the very building block of the many mind-body techniques introduced in this book. Noticing builds self awareness and with greater awareness comes greater choice about how to respond.

Impact On Your Body

First, notice what is happening in your body. When you are distressed your breathing is shallow, your muscles tense and your heart pounds. You might sweat more, develop headaches or stomach aches or suffer from diarrhea or constipation. Each of us holds tension differently in our bodies. Where do you hold yours? In your neck and shoulders? Your chest? Your jaw? Your stomach? Take time to notice precisely where you hold tension and what it feels like. How would you describe the feeling of tension? A throb, a tightness, or clenching? A closing down feeling?

A discomfort or pain? What is the overall impression in your body? A jittery, charged, or restless sensation?

Impact On Your Mind

Distressing thoughts consume a tremendous amount of energy. They are exhausting. They can take on a life of their own and spin out of control. You can feel like you are going crazy. You project yourself into the future and imagine all the things that could go wrong. You drag yourself back into your past and ruminate about all the things that should have happened differently. Perhaps you embroider – adding a new twist to each cycle of the same thought. Your mind goes around and around on these well worn tracks, grieving, worrying, obsessing, "awfulizing" and making yourself miserable.

What do you notice about your mind in this state? Are you able to concentrate and work effectively at the task at hand? Not likely. Instead you are probably operating on a short fuse: snapping at others and flitting from one task to the other with impatience and a diminished attention span.

The distressed mind, like the distressed body, is super charged and restless. Sleep comes in fits and starts; and after several nights of restless sleep, a build-up of fatigue makes everything worse.

Impact On Your Spirit

Are you enjoying your day and the company around you? No. When your mind is filled with distressing thoughts, you are closed to everything else. You are not enjoying the sunrise, or the smell of morning coffee brewing or the opportunities for connection with family, friends or colleagues around you. It could be a lovely day outside, but you won't notice. You are not in the present moment. Your worries have transported you to a miserable existence in the future or in the past and you are missing the moment that is unfolding now. You are missing out on your own life.

You Are Being Hijacked

A young mother in one of our groups perceptively described this as hijacking. What a perfect word to describe how our thoughts hold us hostage and isolate us from people we love:

I was supposed to be playing a board game with my daughter. I didn't even notice it was my turn to move because I was so lost in my worries. My daughter made a joke of it, but I could tell she was disappointed with me. Another time, I was reading to my son and he had to take my head in his little hands to focus me back on the page. I wasn't even aware I had stopped reading. I'm letting my cancer thoughts take over. I'm letting them hijack me from enjoying time with my own children.

Both the story and the term "hijacking" hit an instant chord. Fellow group members immediately identified with the situation. They nodded their heads and told their own stories of being hijacked.

So how are you going to deal with these terrorists? The choice is ultimately yours. Are you going to allow them to hijack you to an unknown future or an imperfect past? Or are you going to respond in different ways, not only to find more peaceful outcomes, but also to give your body the very best chance to heal and get well?

Red Alert

Over time, distressed or worried thoughts can break down the body's natural resilience. Our bodies react to stress with the "fight or flight" stance, a response that is hard wired into our physiology and was necessary for our survival in primitive times when threat came in the form of a hairy mammoth. But now that threats come in the form of distressed and worried thoughts, this stance does not work well for us anymore. In "fight or flight" mode adrenalin pumps into the body – increasing heart rate, blood pressure, blood sugar levels and sweat gland production. Muscles tense, and pupils dilate. In essence, the body is charged and ready for action. But in modern times we rarely fight or flee (as much as we might wish to at times) so this pent up energy is not used. Our bodies stay on "red alert" and overtime this erodes our natural defenses and affects our health and wellbeing.

Five Steps to a Calmer Mind

So far we have established that distressed thoughts create much of our suffering and we have documented the power of their impact on our bodies, minds and spirits. Hopefully it is now abundantly clear that learning to manage our thoughts more effectively can not only reduce much of the suffering that comes with illness, but also create optimal conditions for healing to take place. In this chapter we discuss five steps to a more peaceful mind:

1. Cultivating the inner observer
2. Identifying thoughts
3. Reframing for a more peaceful perspective
4. Discharging restless energy
5. Reinforcing intent

Cultivating the Inner Observer

When some of the old feelings come up, I can be the observer and stay present and calm. It just feels wonderful. My humor is coming back.

The first step in managing your thoughts more effectively is to notice what you are saying to yourself. Can you tell the difference between having a thought and watching yourself have a thought? This is key. Normally you just think. You probably haven't been taught to notice yourself think. The thought comes and goes without you standing back to notice. You are on automatic pilot.

It takes a certain skill and some practice to stand back and notice. The skill requires focused attention. The moment you observe your thought, you break your complete identification with it. You have opened up a space to maneuver. You now have increased your potential to respond differently. You have more control. You are no longer on automatic pilot.

Let's work with an example to make this clearer. Let's say you are waiting to hear the results of a test. You are very anxious about this because you have had some symptoms that suggest to you that the cancer may be growing and you have to wait ten days before the appointment in this state of heightened tension. You ruminate constantly about the nature of the symptoms, what they might mean, the difficulty of waiting to hear, and all the challenges and heartbreaks that are in store for you if the cancer returns. These worries seem constantly with you, like shadows hovering in the background, weaving in and out of your day, making you tense and miserable.

Now imagine you have the ability to stand apart from yourself and observe your own thought stream as it happens. The very act of stepping out to look in gives you some power. You are no longer in your thoughts. You are looking at them. Notice what you are saying to yourself. Identify the worries. For example, you may be saying to yourself in different ways: "I'm frightened the cancer is getting worse. I won't be able to cope. I can't do this anymore. I want the whole thing to stop."

Watching your self have these thoughts is different from having the thoughts. You have removed yourself one step and created an opening. In that opening lies the possibility of responding differently. Instead of being a passive victim to these miserable thoughts, you can work with the space you have created. You can say, "Stop. These thoughts aren't helping me right now. My symptoms could mean a number of different things. I don't need to jump to the worst case scenario. I'm going to choose to think more peaceful thoughts right now."

More examples of reframing troubled thoughts will follow later. The important point here is to develop the skill of watching your thoughts — developing the focused attention you need to monitor your own thought stream. As you practice this, you will become more adept at catching yourself in patterns of thinking that lead you to distress the moment they occur. Then you can say to yourself something like "There's that same thought again. It's making me miserable. I'm not going to do this to myself right now."

You are not stopping your thoughts. You are noticing them. As you notice them, you break your complete immersion in them. You have some space now to respond in different ways other than to passively flow into the misery they create.

In the Healing Journey Program, we call this practice "mind watching." Essentially you are cultivating an Inner Observer, a facility of tuning into your thought stream and exerting this presence to direct your thoughts in a more healing direction.

Developing this focused attention is not as easy as it sounds. We are used to thinking only. We are not used to thinking about thinking. You are probably aware that you are having thoughts that are making you miserable. The challenge is to catch them as you think them.

Even when you do, success is rarely immediate. Telling yourself to think more peaceful thoughts is not going to work instantly. Your mind will respond with impatience. It will quickly return to all the reasons to be miserable and insist on taking you there. This is not a magic formula. The disturbing thought does not immediately go away. It may never go away. But as you develop your Inner Observer, as you become more aware of your thoughts and the impact they have on you, gradually you begin to have some ability to change how you respond to the distressing thought. Do not give up. A little success is all you need to convince you of your power to make a difference. After fifteen years of working with people teaching them these skills, I know, without a doubt, that such practices can make a huge impact.

Two techniques, described in the next chapter, are particularly beneficial in developing mind watching skills: meditation and journaling. Meditation hones your ability to turn inwards and observe the workings of your mind as it unfolds. Over time, as you continue with meditation, you become more and more able to experience this Inner Observer as a calm, spacious presence. Journaling helps you to understand your patterns of behavior and the triggers that cause you to react in ways that culminate in stress. This greater awareness allows you to "mind watch" more effectively and to respond in healthier ways.

Identifying Thoughts

Once you get into the habit of observing your mind, you can tune in regularly to identify the make-up of your thoughts more readily. You can observe your thought stream at different times of day. What is it like when you first wake up in the morning? When you go to bed at night? As you travel to and from work? Tuning in regularly helps you become more aware of what you are saying to yourself at many levels. While the obvious worries may be readily observable to you, sometimes thoughts are more subtle. There may be longstanding patterns of thinking that have come to impact your moods significantly, but because they are so ingrained, you are not aware of them – even when you stop to notice. They move into automatic pilot so quickly they become part of your mental outlook. They are so familiar you don't perceive them separately; they are like faded wallpaper you have lived with for so long you no longer see the shape or pattern. Here is an example:

You Have Cancer. You Can't Be Happy.

Mary came to the Healing Journey program not sure why she had enrolled. She didn't really think about her cancer very much. She expected to complete treatment and resume her old life in short order. She didn't worry much. She kept busy and had several projects on the go to take her mind off the disease. The only time she really thought about cancer was on Wednesday mornings from 10-12 a.m. when she came to our program or when she was receiving treatment. At other times, cancer was the farthest thing from her mind.

Recently she noticed she wasn't enjoying time with her friends very much. This was new. She was impatient when they talked about their lives. She felt frustrated and unhappy and wanted to go home. She expected it was because she was tired from treatment and didn't think much of it. But when questioned by members of the Healing Journey group, she began to recognize that this feeling of unhappiness was more pervasive than she first acknowledged. For example, when she was watching a favorite TV show at home by herself, she'd start off enjoying herself and then something would happen and she'd experience the same restlessness and discontent she experienced with her friends. When she was busy, she was fine, so she kept very busy.

Then Mary did an exercise in mind watching. In this exercise, participants are asked to recall a recent event which had some kind of emotional charge for them. They are asked to imagine that their mind has controls like a video camera so that they can slow down the speed of the memory and zoom in on any part of the memory that carried emotional weight for them. The idea is to become more aware of the thoughts behind the emotions; to develop a skill in which you can stand back and watch your own mind like an observer.

The exercise usually takes several tries before much comes of it. When thoughts are operating on automatic pilot, it is quite difficult to slow them down to observe them. Sometimes people do have startling insights into the workings of their own mind right away and such was the case for Mary. It became clear to her that she was telling herself a central message over and over again without being aware of it. The message was simple, powerful and effective in its crippling way. The message was this: "You have cancer. You can't be happy."

This was the wallpaper she was living in without noticing it. When she was out with friends, when she was home watching TV, when she first woke up in the morning, that message was there lurking at the back of her mind. Keeping busy helped her to avoid it. Saying it out loud paradoxically came as a huge relief. By becoming aware of it, she could begin the work of dismantling it. By slowing down to notice her automatic thinking, she could exert more influence.

Mary's example hits home with many cancer patients and their loved ones. What thoughts do you have on automatic pilot? What are you telling yourself about your cancer or your friend or family member's cancer? How much suffering is it causing you? Is there another way of thinking?

Reframing For a More Peaceful Perspective

Once you are aware of what you are saying to yourself, you can choose to redirect your thoughts toward a more peaceful perspective. Sometimes this involves challenging the validity or truthfulness of the thought. Take Mary's message: "You have cancer. You can't be happy." Is this true? Does a diagnosis of cancer bring an obligation to be miserable? No. Is it possible to be happy, to live a fulfilled life and have cancer? Yes. Mary had only to look around the room to see many examples of people enjoying their lives and living with cancer. The fact a message is irrational doesn't change its power to keep you miserable. Stay alert to such automatic messaging. The next time Mary went out with her friends and felt restless when they started to talk about their vacations or their boyfriends, she recognized the familiar pattern. Instead of feeling unhappy and alone with her cancer in contrast to her friends, she identified the sneaky invader. She could say to herself, "Ah there you are again. I recognize you. Stop. I can have cancer and I can be happy. I'm not going to let this irrational thought take me away from enjoying this moment with my friends."

Mind watching gives you choices. Like Mary, you can move from automatic pilot to your own controls. As a tool to change direction, try imagining a large "Stop" sign in your mind and then deliberately choose different ways of thinking about whatever it is that is preoccupying you. If it is hard for you to visualize a Stop sign, try repeating the word "Stop" emphatically to yourself. Another practice some people use effectively is to wear an elastic band around their wrists. Every time they notice an upsetting thought, they pull the band and let it snap back against their wrists. The action acts as a Stop sign for them, signaling the need to halt, take a deep breath and reframe the thought.

Another tool to redirect distressful thoughts is to return to the present moment. We have already noted how thoughts are like hijackers taking us away from what is happening around us. Tell yourself to stop the distressing thought and focus instead on what is presently happening. Appreciate and enjoy your life as it is presently unfolding. Some people make a pact with their thoughts. They acknowledge the distressing thoughts and set a time to deal with them later. This frees them to continue their day, without the worries, until the appointed time.

What Happens if the Distressing Thoughts are True?

Often troubling thoughts have some truth to them.

I'm worried this chemo will make me sick and miserable like last time.

The doctor who misdiagnosed me let me down.

My husband isn't supporting me when I need him.

I should have stopped smoking.

I should have listened to my gut feeling and sought help earlier.

The odds are against me.

In these cases, it is important to recognize that you are making yourself miserable by constantly repeating distressing thoughts to yourself. Do you want to continue doing this? Can you see that you have a choice? Is there another gentler way of framing these thoughts? Perhaps it would be helpful to review the common worries and fears described in chapter one and look at how others reframed these thoughts in more hopeful ways.

One strategy that has worked for many is to repeat again and again to yourself the following:

I choose peace. Not this. I choose peace. Not this.

Try it and you may be surprised how quickly it works to bring you to a calmer place. Use it repeatedly and the comfort of these words can act as a sanctuary from distress bringing calm and solace to the restless mind. You can use it anywhere, at any time you are upset: when someone cuts in on you in your car; when a colleague annoys you at work; when a family member gets on your nerves; when worries about cancer take over your mind. Notice your distress, take a deep breath and repeat, "I choose peace. Not this."

Another phrase that is very effective for many and helps in those moments of physical or emotional pain or when the present moment is uncomfortable in anyway, is to repeat like a mantra:

This too, shall pass. This too, shall pass.

As difficult as the moment may be, pain comes and goes. This is true for both emotional and physical pain. Nothing lasts forever. When things are really unbearable, take solace in the fact the difficult situation won't last. Remember that there is always opportunity for hope and hope means different things at different times. There is always the possibility of opening yourself to greater comfort, and finding warmth within. As remote and elusive as this may seem at times, it may help to know that whatever you are experiencing will pass with time.

When Reframing Doesn't Work

Sometimes our distressing thoughts are linked to strong feelings that cannot easily be redirected or reframed toward more peaceful perspectives. There may be too much hurt, anger, shame, grief or bitterness at the root of them. That's okay. Healing is a process. It takes time. Thoughts related to hurt or angry feelings lodge deeply and stubbornly into consciousness and are not reframed in a convincing way very easily.

How do you move through anger and hurt? It takes determination, patience and practice. It can be done. We will discuss this in more detail later in the book when we discuss the troubled heart, letting go and particularly forgiveness. Forgiveness of self and others is a very powerful healing tool.

For the moment, it is enough to begin. Start by noticing the impact on your body, mind and spirit. Re-read the earlier paragraphs on this subject and identify how it applies to you. How does holding onto your anger and hurt affect you at each of these levels? If the anger and hurt are constantly looping around the same well rutted cycles and eat away at you constantly, you are sacrificing peacefulness in mind, body and spirit in service of this obsession. It is in your best interests to find a way through this. Staying stuck in anger and hurt helps no one. This is the core work of warming the troubled heart and the subject of chapters four and five. Ultimately moving through anger and hurt requires letting go of the hold these thoughts and feelings have over you and opening your heart to handle them in different ways.

Discharging Restless Energy

As we have noted, distress brings restless energy into our bodies. We are agitated and we feel this charge at every level: a racing pulse, jangled nerves, tense muscles, sweaty glands and upset stomach. We are on red alert and we are wired to fight or flee. We have lost our calm and often we have also lost our balance and perspective.

What do you do with this restless energy? When your body and mind feel charged by restless and disturbing thoughts? I regularly ask this question in the Healing Journey Program when we talk about calming the mind. One of the most memorable answers was given by a young woman who said she closed all the curtains in her home, then put on the Rolling Stones full blast and danced nude around her house, completely losing herself in the music. Another answer that has stayed with me over the years is one given by a married couple who would wake up in the middle of the night, both stirred by worries and fears related to her ovarian cancer. They would each head to their laptop computers and sit side- by-side at a long table to write about their worried thoughts and feelings. They found solace in writing and companionship in doing it together. Most often they did not share with each other what they had written. They respected their need for private outlets. A common list of more typical answers might look like this:

- Go for a jog, bike, swim
- Talk to a trusted friend who is a good listener
- Write in a journal
- Dance
- Sing

- Build something
- Go shopping
- Practice Yoga, Tai Chi, or Chi Gong
- Immerse in work
- Have a good cry
- Chant
- Walk the beach
- Let off steam in the shower: scream, yell, sing
- Meditate
- Pray
- Commune with a cat, dog, horse
- Drum
- Commune with nature
- Paint; draw; splash colors
- Knit
- Play musical instrument

You will know which of these outlets works for you. Usually they help for a while to calm the mind and reduce restless energy. In addition, learning and practicing breathing and relaxation exercises are critical to redirecting your body, mind and spirit toward greater calm and wellbeing. Such practices are powerful, effective and well researched. They are described in the next chapter.

Reinforcing Intent

Our tendency is to slip back into old habits. This is particularly true of thinking habits. If our thoughts tend toward worry and turmoil, we have to regularly check in with ourselves to notice when our automatic pilot has led us once again down those well rutted routes. We have to regularly reinforce our intention to steer toward more peaceful pathways. Several factors reinforce this intent: belief you can do it; patience; and a gentle open perspective.

Belief: "I Can Do It"

Do you believe it is possible to change how you think? When I raise this question, I think of Lucy. Lucy came to the Healing Journey program because her husband had cancer and she needed support. Typically couples come together, but sometimes one partner has no interest in coming or is too busy or sick to participate. Lucy was dealing with a difficult situation. Her husband was in hospital and Lucy wanted to be there as much as she could to ensure he got the care he needed. But her immediate and extended family needed her at home and everyone relied on Lucy to sort out multiple problems and make things better. Each week, Lucy came to the group with new problems involving incompetent care of her husband and the overwhelming demands on her to solve those problems, keep the house tidy, meals on the table and generally respond to the needs and cares of others around her. Such was the toll on her, she could not sleep and she had trouble sitting still throughout the group session. She often arrived late or left early because of time pressures. She had no time for herself and the strain was debilitating.

Fellow group members identified with many of the things she described. They applauded her care for her husband and family and empathized with the many challenges she faced. They were concerned about the evident cost to her wellbeing and how much responsibility she shouldered alone. Some talked about how they had to learn to accept help from others and to not "sweat the small stuff" like having a perfectly tidy house or winning every family argument on chores and responsibilities. So what if the house was untidy and the laundry didn't get done? Let someone else deal with it for once. But Lucy had exacting standards and could not rely on anyone but herself for the many tasks she encountered at home and at the hospital. She refused all offers of help from family and friends because it took too long to explain what was needed and it was easier to do it herself.

After weeks of such stories, a fellow group member said emphatically, "Lucy, you're wearing yourself out. You need to accept help from others." Lucy welcomed the comment. She proceeded to document all the reasons why it was impossible to rely on anyone else but herself. Underneath everything she reported was the thought: "It's all up to me. If I don't do it, everything will fall apart." This is the central message she kept telling herself.

At this point, I asked her to stop and look at her automatic thinking and how it contributed to her feelings of stress. She agreed she was constantly telling herself "It's all up to me" whether it was managing her husband's care, looking after the house or solving problems for the family. She could also see that she added to this pressure by imagining worse case scenarios if she didn't immediately step in and solve things. She knew these thoughts created much of her distress but she remained unconvinced there was anything she could do about it.

The group then talked generally about the challenge of managing stressful situations and the difficulty of changing thought patterns. When I asked them was it even possible to change how we think, Lucy answered with a resounding and feisty, "No!" We all laughed, mostly because we needed a light intervention at that point. We also laughed because it was a relief to find the crux of the matter: What we believe shapes how we think and how we act.

I appreciated Lucy's response because her vibrant "No" highlights the difficulties involved in re-orienting our thinking toward more peaceful avenues. It is not easy. At times, we all feel like yelling a resounding, "No" – the effort of reframing and looking at things differently seems to ask too much. There is comfort in our old cycles of thinking, even if they do take us down troubled pathways.

However, if we begin to have some experiences of success, we know we have power to effect change. Even if for only a moment, on one or two occasions, we are successful in noticing and reframing our worried or fearful thoughts, then we know we can exert some control. We know it is possible, at least some of the time. And that belief is all powerful. That experience gives substance to the belief, that yes, we can do it: we can purposively move our thinking toward peace of mind.

Patience

Most of us are hard on ourselves: we expect a lot. So if we don't immediately succeed at channeling worried thoughts into more peaceful directions, we think we are no good at it, and give up. I can't say this often enough: it is not easy to change the way we think. It is okay to struggle with it. Pretty well everyone does. Wherever you are in the process is just fine. Sometimes you will find you can bring your mind to a more peaceful place; sometimes you won't. Some days things will come easily; you will feel joyous and peaceful; other days you will feel as if despair trails you like a pervasive fog and there is no way out. Everything looks and feels bleak. That's okay too. It is natural to have days like that from time to time. It only becomes a problem if your thoughts stay stuck in that bleak place for an extended time. So be patient with yourself when nothing seems to work and you feel discouraged, frightened and alone. Most often these days will pass and you will find yourself feeling better again and ready to resume your intent to direct your thoughts in more peaceful directions.

Gentleness/Kindness

Closely related to being patient with yourself is being gentle with yourself. As you become more adept at watching your thought stream, you will likely notice a steady stream of judgments about yourself and others. Most of us have highly critical thought streams. For greater peace of mind, it is not only important to notice what we are saying to ourselves about our cancer, it is also important to notice what we are saying to ourselves about ourselves, and others. Be alert to subtle and not so subtle messages about not measuring up in some way. The following excerpt was written by a middle-aged man who was well aware of the pervasive and crippling effect of such thoughts:

I seem to be afraid to start or attempt anything for fear of failure or looking foolish. As long as I can remember, I'm afraid I may do something wrong, or may fail in my attempt thereby making myself look foolish or stupid. It's emotionally draining. Despite all the encouragement I get from the group and my family and friends, I continue in this pattern.

Here is the best reason for being gentle with yourself: you are your own most powerful tool in dealing with the turmoil cancer brings to your life. Strength, courage and vitality to live fully no matter what you face are dependent on your own inner resources. Your inner resources will work best if they are fueled by kind encouragement rather than impatient criticism. Treat yourself as you would a beloved and sometimes vulnerable good friend or young child. We all make mistakes. We are all vulnerable and fallible at times. Watch the lens through which you view yourself and others. Foster kindness to yourself.

Practice, Practice, Practice . . .

To really make a difference, you will need to practice what you have learned. Tune into your thoughts several times a day. When you are distressed, try and catch your thoughts as you think them. Identify the central message you are telling yourself. As you notice or catch your thoughts, you break your complete identification with them. In this space you have some room to maneuver: to reframe your thoughts in ways more conducive to peace and wellbeing. Discharge restless energy by engaging in activities that feel right for you and by practicing breathing and relaxation exercises. Do this again and again, reinforcing your intent to calm your mind. When you slip back into old habits, be patient and kind with yourself. The next chapter will build upon and reinforce these steps toward a calmer mind.

Three
Five Techniques
to Calm your Mind and Body

1. **Breath Awareness**
2. **Mind/Body Relaxation**
3. **Meditation**
4. **Guided Imagery**
5. **Journaling**

Reading about calming your mind is not enough. This chapter gives you information and instructions on how to get a healing practice established, personalized and integrated in your life so that more of your day is spent in a peaceful state of mind. The more you practice, the more powerful and reliable these techniques become for you.

At first taking the time to try out these practices can seem like a chore. If you're like most people, you won't want to do it: instead you will want to escape from the turmoil of the day and your circumstances into watching TV or some other activity that helps you to forget everything for a while. It is totally understandable. However, try to get past thinking of these techniques as chores and instead view them as opportunities for healing: time with yourself for some peace and quiet. So much is guided by our mindset – if we think something's going to be a chore, it usually is one. A certain amount of willpower and discipline is needed in order to stick to doing these practices long enough to experience their benefits. If you find the experience frustrating at first, you are not alone. It does take time and commitment on your part to get past the initial frustration and skepticism.

"Making It Real"

How can you use these techniques so they make a difference in your life? That's the crux of the matter. We are not aiming for momentary experiences of peacefulness, as welcome as they might be. We are aiming for changes that make an experiential difference in your day-to-day life.

"Making it Real" was coined by Nancy, a vibrant middle aged woman living with pancreatic cancer. She used the expression to convey the idea that the important part of her practice was not doing the techniques or discussing her evolving sense of healing, but feeling the practice and living the understanding so that her life was transformed. She also called this "living the revelation."

It's not enough to do the practices, you have to live it, feel it, personalize it. You have to make it real to yourself.

Feeling Right

Personalized meaning transforms experience. It grows out of a "feeling right" experience – a sense that the practice resonates deeply in your mind, body and spirit. This "feeling right" quality may be very subtle at first: a momentary sense of opening or peacefulness or a kind of "Ahhhh" relief feeling. Or the "feeling right" quality may be very strong and have an instant impact – like being overtaken by a rush of feeling, a wave of peacefulness, or a powerful sense of being loved and cared for.

Whether the "feeling right" quality is mild or strong or any-where in-between, it will certainly pass – as all emotional states eventually do. This is where "making it real" comes into play. Notice and believe in the impact you have experienced. Continue to practice the technique so that it becomes second nature to you. Make use of the experience, when you can, in your day-to-day life. Here are some examples that will illustrate what I mean.

Louise struggled with meditation. She set aside time to do it daily and practiced for 15 minutes every day for a week. But she found her mind remained very busy and the exercise felt like a chore. She did not stick with it. "It just didn't seem to fit with me." But then a fellow group member suggested meditating on the prayer of St. Francis. Although she was not religious, she decided to give it a try. She was very surprised to find the prac-tice clicked instantly. "I don't know why but it brought me a feeling of calm – almost a "coming home" feeling. After that meditation had meaning for me. It was no longer a chore."

Sarah woke from a dream in which she imagined herself surrounded by angels singing a hymn. In the dream she experienced a tremendous feeling of warmth and compassion and when she woke she continued to sing the hymn in order to maintain this wonderful feeling of care and connection. From then on, she used the hymn as a way of bringing feelings of peace and calm into her day.

Small Steps

What if nothing resonates? It is hard to hear personal stories of peace and healing when nothing is working for you or when you miss out on experiences others seem to have. Remember the central tenet of this book is that wherever you are in your process is just fine. From any point, there is always the possibility of moving toward greater comfort and peace. The Chinese philosopher Confucius said, "A journey of a 1000 miles begins with a single step."

By reading this book, you have already taken a single step. Don't worry if you have no 'feeling right' experiences. Trust the process. Practice the techniques and hone your ability to notice your own experience. With time and practice, the routine is likely to bring you feelings of peacefulness and calm. Notice them, enjoy them, relax into them. They will pass. But even a momentary experience or glimmer into the feelings of a relaxed body and mind will be enough for you to know it is possible to experience them. It won't happen every time you practice. Some days nothing seems to work. But as you maintain your routine, you create a space for such experiences to happen. Gradually, over time they become more consistently a part of your practice.

Establishing a routine

- Try each of the five techniques
- Which works or "feels right"?
- Develop and personalize practice
- Practice at least 20 minutes daily
- "Make it real": feel, live, practice meaningfully
- Bring yourself back to your practice when you fall away

Don't be hard on yourself; for most of us, it takes time to establish a routine

More and more, bring peaceful awareness into your day to day living

1. Breath Awareness

I got bad news today. I started to panic and then I reminded myself, "breathe, just breathe."

What is Breath Awareness?

It is bringing your mind to focus on your breathing, as you breathe in and as you breathe out. It is the simplest and most important technique you can learn to quiet your body and mind. Breath awareness is the cornerstone of mind-body techniques, such as yoga, tai chi, chi gong, relaxation and meditation. Eastern thought equates the flow of breath with the flow of life force through the body. Breath work, then, is an important component of health, wellness and spirit.

How Can It Help Me?

In a moment of anxiety or sudden emotion, it can give you some space from the sudden grip of feeling. Focusing on your breath in meditation can bring mental calmness and peaceful expansiveness. Being aware of your breath helps you to be mindful, alert and joyful in the present moment.

I notice more when I'm getting emotional. I sense – "I'm going to lose it. I'm going to lose it." I feel emotion well up in me. I stop and step away from it. I breathe deeply. It helps.

Try It

Close your eyes and notice your breathing. Bring your full attention to following your breath as you inhale and as you exhale. Try not to judge; simply observe what you find.

What Do You Notice?

Whatever you notice is fine. You are not trying to consciously control your breath in any way or achieve any particular result.

The practice is about training your mind to notice and sustain attention of the breath. As you become more comfortable with the practice, you will find the quality of your breath naturally changes, becoming slower, deeper, more rhythmic and peaceful.

Relaxing Breath: Deep Breathing

Now try this. Sit comfortably making sure your back is straight so your lungs can breathe fully and easily. Close your eyes. Breathe in deeply through your nose. As you breathe in, your belly softly rises. Then breathe out through your mouth, pushing out as much air as you comfortably can. Your belly contracts softly inward. The key to deep breathing is breathing from the abdomen, not the upper chest. If you place your hands on your abdomen you will feel the gentle rising and falling of your belly as you breathe in and out. Most of us tend to take shallow breaths in and out from our chest area. Certainly when we are tense, our breathing is shallow. By learning to breathe from our abdomens again (babies do this automatically), we are bringing more oxygen into our bodies and learning to relax and refresh ourselves.

Breathe in Comfort; Breathe Out Tension

As you breathe in, imagine breathing in comfort and imagine this comfort flooding through your body like a healing energy. Imagine breathing in warmth, light, and healing. Imagine breathing in kindness, love and care. Then as you breathe out, bring a "letting go" quality to the out breath. You might even say "Ahhhhh" as you breathe out to encourage the release of tension in your body and worries from your mind. With each out breath, comes the opportunity to release a little bit more of the daily tensions we all tend to carry in our bodies most of the time. With each cycle of your breath, you are breathing in comfort and breathing out tension. Allow yourself to relax into the comforting rhythm of your breath. Allow yourself to relax more and more with each cycle of your breath.

"Breathing In, I Calm My Body. Breathing Out, I Smile."

This is a manta suggested by Thich Nhat Hanh – -a Vietnamese Buddhist monk, who has written many books on finding inner peace and meaning. [A mantra is a repetitive focus on peaceful words to calm the mind.] As you inhale, you repeat to yourself, "Breathing in, I calm my body" and as you exhale, "Breathing out, I smile." When you smile, your body automatically relaxes a little. Imagine the feeling of a smile moving through your entire body from the top of your head to your feet. Repeating these words to yourself can be very soothing and relaxing.

Practice. Practice. Practice.

Tune into your breath many times throughout the day to calm and refresh yourself at work or at home. Practice mindful breathing to bring yourself back to the present moment in a fully engaged way. In a moment of tension, breathe deeply to give yourself a moment of space and to help calm your mind and body. Practice breathing in comfort and breathing out tension so the process becomes familiar and comfortable for you. We will be building on these skills as we learn the next techniques in this chapter and chapter six.

Further Practice and Study

As breath awareness is central to relaxation and meditation, you will get lots more practice with developing this capacity as we move through this book and as you begin to transform your life toward peacefulness away from distraction and despair.

2 . Mind/Body Relaxation

I am reaching a deeper relaxed state with regular practice.

My breathing seems to be deeper and slower. I have a "letting go"'feeling. It's warm and calming.

I can alter things in my life: I can put a floor on my down periods. Those are more controllable through imagery and relaxation.

Mind/Body Connection

You can calm your mind by relaxing your body. The two go together. It is pretty difficult to have a stressed mind and a relaxed body. Think about that for a moment. The connection is important. If you cannot redirect your thoughts in more peaceful directions, you can still overcome mental distress by focusing on your body instead of your mind. If you can learn to relax your body, your mind automatically follows suit.

What is Mind/Body Relaxation?

It is a state of relaxed body and calm mind. Your body is comfortable, open and at ease and your mind is quiet and restful. There are several forms of relaxation training. All build on breath awareness, the easy rise and fall of inhalation and exhalation. Two techniques are introduced here – deep muscle relaxation, which involves active tensing and relaxing different muscle groups throughout the body and deep inner relaxation, which involves scanning your body and imagining your body progressively softening and easing and becoming more comfortable.

How Can It Help Me?

A relaxed body and mind give the body its best chance for healing. It is self evident that optimal conditions for recovery are more likely associated with relaxation than distress. Research shows relaxation training lowers blood pressure, slows breathing and heart rates, increases blood flow and relieves chronic pain and symptoms of anxiety and depression.

As training deepens, you will not only become more relaxed, you will also more readily identify when you are feeling tense in your day-to-day life. Just as you have learned to regularly tune into your thought stream, you can regularly scan your body for tension. With this awareness, you will be more able to identify stress throughout the day and make appropriate adjustments. As you relax your body, you calm your mind.

Getting Ready

Find a quiet place. Loosen any tight clothing, take off your shoes. Turn off phones and free yourself from other distractions. Give yourself permission to take this time for relaxation without interruptions, worries and doubts. Create an inner space for relaxation to occur – be open to the experience and easy with yourself.

Try It: Deep Muscle Relaxation

This involves actively tensing and releasing different muscle groups in your body. The goal is for you to notice what your muscles feel like when they are tense and relaxed and what the difference is between the two. If you have places of tenderness or soreness in your body – often the case after surgery or treatment, skip this technique and proceed to the next one – deep inner relaxation. Only engage in actively tensing your muscles if it is comfortable to do so.

- **Bring awareness to your breath:** Breathe in and out, slowly and deeply as you did in the first exercise. Breathe in comfort, breathe out tension. You might like to say "Ahhh" as you breathe out to encourage the release of stress in your body and mind. Spend several minutes relaxing into your breath cycle before you begin the muscle tensing and releasing sequence. Continue to breathe comfortably and deeply throughout the exercise.

- **Hands:** Make a tight fist with your right hand, clenching the fingers and studying the tension. Hold it, then release. Notice the difference. Repeat. Now try it with your left hand and repeat. Let the tension drain away completely. Next clench both hands at once, then release. Feel the difference – your hands are now open and relaxed.

- **Arms:** Make fists and lift them up to your shoulders as if you are lifting weights. Feel the tension, hold it, then let it go. Always notice the difference. Now try the opposite movement – pushing your arms away from your body. Relax and repeat.

- **Shoulders:** Lift your shoulders up to your ears, using the same sequence of tensing, holding, noticing, releasing and paying attention to the difference. Repeat.

- **Neck:** gently bring your chin down to your chest, feeling the pull of muscles at the back of your neck. Hold and release. Now tilt your head slightly to one side, then the other. Notice the tension, let it go, feel the difference.

- **Face:** Raise your eyebrows to the top of your forehead. Release. Now bring your eyebrows together, creasing your forehead into a frown. Release. Clench your jaw and force a smile. Relax. Purse your lips together in disapproval, then let go. Make a prune face scrunching your face up to your nose. Release. Let your whole face relax. Feel the softness. Repeat the sequence.

Chest: Take a deep breath and hold it. Notice the tension in the chest area and release. Repeat. Remember to continue breathing deeply and comfortably throughout the exercise.

Stomach: Take a deep breath in and tense the muscles in your stomach. Imagine you are preparing yourself for a punch. Hold the tension and then let it go. Repeat.

Back: Gently arch your back outward making a small movement. Feel the tension then release. Repeat.

Legs and feet: Tense your buttocks and thighs by pressing down onto your heels. Hold, release and repeat. Now press down on your toes feeling the tension in your shins and calves. Hold, release and repeat. Notice the difference.

Scan your body and relax into your breathing. Check the body for any remaining tension and let it go. Let a relaxed feeling wash over your body, mind and spirit. Relax into your breathing.

Finish by imagining yourself in a very peaceful place. Picture yourself there with all your senses: seeing, hearing, feeling, touching and smelling all the peaceful components of this special place. [Greater detail is given in technique# 4—guided imagery.] Let the last vestiges of tension slip from your body and mind and relax deeply into comfort and peace.

Try it: Deep Inner Relaxation

This exercise also involves scanning your body, but instead of actually tensing and releasing your muscles, you imagine them becoming more relaxed by encouraging feelings of warmth, heaviness, and comfort. You need to actively engage your imagination to make this exercise real and powerful for yourself. Find out by trial and error which suggestions or images work most effectively for you.

- **Bring awareness to your breath**: breathe in and out, slowly and deeply as you did in the first exercise. Breathe in comfort, breathe out tension. You might like to say "Ahhh" as you breathe out to encourage the release of stress in your body and mind. Spend several minutes relaxing into your breath cycle before you begin scanning your body. Continue to breathe comfortably and deeply throughout the exercise.

- **Scan your body:** Imagine a warm healing energy entering into your body through the top of your head, then moving to temples, forehead, around your eyes, cheeks, mouth and jaw. Now the warm healing energy moves down the back of your head, down your neck and spreads across your shoulders. The feeling builds and radiates through your shoulders, down your arms and into your hands and fingers. Perhaps you feel a tingly sensation as the relaxation moves into your hands and fingers.

  Now the warm healing energy moves into the large muscles of your back, and you can feel the warmth flowing down your spine, vertebrae to vertebrae, then into your hips and buttocks. Next the warm healing energy moves into your chest area, through your heart and lungs, and then deeply into your belly, so your belly feels soft and warm. The healing energy spreads through all the organs in your lower body, through your groin and down your legs, along your feet until the last remaining tension just drifts away through the tips of your toes.

- **Really feel each area** as you focus on it: bring active awareness to each body part as if you are in your body. Imagine each area warming, softening, easing, loosening, opening, and becoming more comfortable. Which words or suggestions relax you the most? Experiment with different images to relax and open your body. Besides a warm healing energy, try a beautiful healing light or the flow of nectar or honey to encourage a warm, heavy relaxed feeling. A beautiful color might work too or the feel of a gentle caress. For some areas – neck and shoulders, for example – you might imagine yourself in a warm shower and feel the warm water gently soothing and massaging your tired neck and shoulder muscles so that they are loose and relaxed and at ease.

- **Surrender to the drift of relaxation** as you move through your body. Let go more and more. Remember to keep breathing deeply and relax into the comforting cycle of your breath, breathing in comfort, breathing out tension.

- **Finish by imagining yourself in a very peaceful place.** Picture yourself there with all your senses: seeing, hearing, feeling, touching and smelling all the peaceful components of this special place. [Greater detail is given in technique number four – guided imagery.] Let the last vestiges of tension slip from your body and mind and relax deeply into comfort and peace.

Practice. Practice. Practice.

The more often you do them, the more effective these techniques will become for you. As you deepen your practice, not only will you experience greater relaxation and consistency of effect, but also you will likely be able to do a shortened version anywhere and anytime. Your body will respond readily to the now familiar cues so you need only close your eyes, take a few deep breaths, and imagine a warm healing energy to bring comfort and relaxation throughout your body. Take a few moments at different times in the day to check your body for tension. Become more aware of where you typically hold tension, what it feels like and how to let it go.

Relaxation exercises do get easier with practice. It is also much more enjoyable and beneficial. I can now easily get into a relaxed state and become centred. It is nice to be able to do this whenever I have the opportunity, without a great deal of effort

When I do a relaxation tape, I can literally feel the tension drain from my body. Afterwards I feel more positive and hopeful. I am more able to sort out my feelings, especially if I'm angry or upset. I am able to see things in a different perspective which makes dealing with situations easier. I find it easier to relax the more I practice.

Further Practice and Study

There are many excellent relaxation scripts and CDs you can use to deepen and vary your practice. MP3 players allow instant accessibility: at home or work, while waiting for an appointment, or in transit. Free Healing Journey audio scripts can be downloaded from www.healingjourney.ca. Also recommended are Eli Bay CDs, available through Amazon.com or elibay.com. For further reference on relaxation, read Herbert Benson's books, *The Relaxation Response* and *Timeless Healing*.

3. Meditation

The taut violin string in my head has relaxed.

The meditation left me with a feeling of bliss, absolute peacefulness and happiness. I felt at one with the universe, the discomfort in my hip and neck gone for the moment, leaving me alone with the warmth and beauty of the chant, my breathing slow and easy. From time to time I found myself switching back to my first mantra, "Breathing in, I calm my body. Breathing out, I smile."

Ten minutes of chanting "Om" can get me into a space that changes the way I feel.

What is It?

Meditation is a way of quieting the mind through focused awareness. The body is relaxed and the mind is alert. It is an active process of bringing the mind to concentrate on a particular focus – such as the breath, a word, an image, a chant, a prayer or series of movements. Over time this practice brings deep inner calm and expansive awareness.

What Is the Experience Like?

As you start, you attend fully to your breath, or another focus of your choice. But then your mind is distracted by thoughts, feelings, or sensations. So the practice becomes noticing the distraction and gently bringing your attention back to the breath. You do this again and again as your mind repeatedly wanders. Untrained minds are naturally restless, jumping from thought to thought like unruly monkeys leaping from tree to tree. As you continue in your meditation practice, you experience moments of calm and peacefulness. Eventually the practice brings inner quiet, comfort and a sense of expansiveness. But all this takes time. An attitude of openness and acceptance to whatever the session brings is the best way to facilitate the gradual deepening of experience.

My mind reminds me of a slippery object which keeps eluding a first grasp. When I try to quiet it, it continually looks for some excuse to run off in some direction or other. It seizes upon any random noise to distract it from silence. Thoughts of current or future events pop into my head, taking me off on tangents and leaving the "quiet" of meditation far behind.

I feel peaceful, round, no edges, almost out of body. Just by staying with my breath, following it, I move into this peaceful space.

Meditation has done a lot for me. In those moments of peace, I feel I'm getting closer to the secret – the meaning of life.

Meditation helps to create space that feels uncluttered.

Meditation has brought me closer to who I am, not who I thought I was supposed to be. Everyone in the family has noticed the difference in me. The more I meditate, the calmer I am.

How Does It Help?

The benefits of meditation are increasingly recognized in western medical journals and include lower blood pressure, better concentration, relief of chronic pain, reduced symptoms of anxiety and depression, improved immune parameters and greater happiness.

A 1980 study by Meares, an Australian psychiatrist, looked at the effects of prolonged meditation, (two hours daily), on 73 cancer patients living with advanced illness. This study was based on anecdotal observation by Meares, not an established research protocol, so the remarkable findings need to be viewed cautiously, but five cancer patients showed complete remission of disease, another five showed marked slowing of cancer growth and most showed improvements in quality of life and significant relief in suffering. Recent research shows that even people who have just learned to meditate and have only been practicing for eight weeks show measurable changes in brain and immune function compared to non-meditators. This is described in more detail in chapter five.

Getting Ready

Find a quiet place. Turn phones off and make sure you won't be interrupted. Sit comfortably with your back straight. Let go of any thoughts or concerns about what meditation is like and what you hope to achieve. In other words, be open to the experience and easy with yourself. Set a timer for 15 or 20 minutes. It helps to practice at the same time every day.

Try it: Focusing On Your Breath

- Close your eyes. (You can leave them open if you prefer. Most people find concentration easier with closed eyes.)
- As you breathe in, bring full attention to observing your breath as it moves into your body.
- As you breathe out, bring full attention to observing your breath as it leaves your body
- If you like, you can count one as you breathe in and one as you breathe out and so on until you reach ten. Then start from one again.
- When your mind wanders, gently bring your attention back to following your breath, as you breathe in and out.
- Continue for 15 minutes; build over time to 30 minutes or longer.
- Sit quietly for a moment or two afterwards before returning to your day.
- Do it every day.

Try it: Focusing On a Word or Phrase (Mantra):

- Pick a focus word, prayer or short phrase that feels right for you, such as "peace," "one" or "be still." If you have a religious or spiritual connection, you may want to consider "Om," "Allah," "Shalom" or "the Lord is my shepherd."
- Close your eyes (or leave them open if you prefer) and breathe slowly and naturally.
- Repeat your focus word silently to yourself as you breathe out.
- When your mind wanders, gently bring your attention back to your focus word.
- Continue for 15 minutes; build over time to 30 minutes or longer.
- Sit quietly for a moment or two afterwards before returning to your day.
- Do it every day.

Try It: Focusing On an Image

- Pick a focus image, such as a candle, flower, picture or symbol.
- Breathe slowly and naturally.
- Bring your full attention to concentrate on the image.
- When your mind wanders, gently bring your focus back to the image.
- Continue for 15 minutes; build over time to 30 minutes or longer.
- Sit quietly for a moment or two afterwards before returning to your day.
- Do it every day.

Nothing's Happening. Am I Doing It Right?

Most people are frustrated or puzzled by their first experiences of meditation. Sitting still and following the breath (or other focus) feels like a waste of time. We are used to being busy and doing many things at once. Success is measured by getting things done and meditation does not fit very easily into that paradigm.

I tried meditating for about 15 minutes a day for a week. I found it very difficult to quiet my mind and I found the practice quite frustrating which is probably why I didn't stick with it.

I'm a doer so I have a hard time sitting still.

Nothing Much is Happening. I Don't Know if I'm Doing It Right

The simple answer to "Am I doing it right?" is yes. If you are sitting quietly and bringing your mind to focus on your breath then you are "doing it right." While the instructions are simple, the practice is difficult. It is not easy to sit quietly and maintain focused concentration. Be patient. Try to stick to meditation long enough to appreciate its benefits.

I used to think if I didn't still my mind in meditation, it wasn't a success. I don't look at it that way anymore. I've learned it doesn't help. The meditation is what it is — which is a very difficult thing to explain to someone. I take some time and I create some space and I am there with myself.

Afterwards I feel more contented. I'm able to deal with some things a little bit better; stresses are a little bit easier to handle. I sense there is a much fuller existence, a much more satisfying life, free of the baggage I carry around in turmoil.

Establishing a Routine:

Meditation practice is helped along by a regular time and place. You can make your own "altar" by bringing personally meaningful items into your meditation space, such as pictures, flowers, candles, incense and peaceful colors. Talking to family members to gain their understanding and support also helps you to stick to your routine. When you fall away from regular practice, bring yourself back to it without guilt or recrimination.

People say they don't have the time, but I make the time. My job is healing. Nothing else is important. That's my main goal in life. Meditation, journaling, Chi-gong, these are the things I'm doing for me. They bring me peace and calmness. When I get the least bit uptight, I just go into calmness. My job is to get me into a healing spot. Meditation keeps me on keel. If I don't do it in the morning, I get more anxious in my day. The more I meditate, the better I am at not holding onto things. I get so much out of it. I wouldn't want to not do it.

Most days I meditate three times a day. I get up in the morning and meditate and then do yoga. I meditate again around three pm and again in the evening. I do imagery all the time. My routine is very healing for me.

I have a special place in my house where I meditate. But I can now meditate anywhere – in my backyard, in my shower and in the car when someone else is driving.

Things work best for me when I take that time to meditate daily. But I don't do it consistently.

I have lapsed for weeks after doing meditation daily for months. Something comes up to upset the routine. It's so easy to slip back into old patterns. I've learned not to feel guilty because that will make it worse.

It's a nice feeling to know I can meditate anywhere. I can get to that peaceful place much faster now. Today, I stayed there for 45 minutes. It felt like heaven.

In the beginning it all seemed very strange to me but as I practice meditating I find that I go "deeper" into myself and become very peaceful, light – almost like I'm floating above

*my body. When I finish with the meditation the peace and
light feeling remain and I feel free to do just about anything.*

Further Practice and Study

There are many more meditation techniques to explore. A
loving kindness meditation is described in chapter six. *Meditation
for Dummies* by Stephan Bodian provides a comprehensive sur-
vey of the range of techniques and tips for starting, maintaining
and deepening meditation. Joining a meditation group in your
community is an excellent way to advance your practice and
build community.

4. Guided Imagery

*My peaceful place is a canoe ride at dawn. It relaxes me
immediately.*

*I picture an expansive sea and sky – it gives me a power-
ful feeling of oneness, of no boundaries, of peace.*

Imagine

Imagine you could take yourself to a very peaceful place
whenever you liked. What location would you choose? A warm
sandy beach? A cottage by a lake? A beautiful waterfall? A pris-
tene mountain top? The fact is you can. All you need do is close
your eyes and imagine yourself there with all your senses.
Guided imagery can take you there as effectively as an airplane.

What is Guided Imagery?

For this exercise, guided imagery is the process of summon-
ing images you can see, hear, feel, smell or taste to create feelings of peace and harmony in your body, mind and spirit. Guided
imagery has wider scope and usage in sports, arts, business,
personal growth and health. Such applications are based on findings that mental imaging can enhance goal setting, creativity
and performance. Imagery is also an effective tool in exploring
deeper thoughts and feelings outside of our everyday awareness.

Isn't It Just Pretend?

While the images are imagined, their effects are real. Your body doesn't discriminate between images in your mind and reality. So imagining an event can have the same impact on the body as experiencing the real event. It may be more muted than experiencing the real event, but the same general physiological response occurs. For example, think about sexual arousal or reliving an angry incident in your mind. Your body responds to the imagined event in the same way as the real event. You can use this to your advantage. By imagining yourself in a peaceful place, your body will relax in the same way as if you were actually there.

There is no scientific proof that guided imagery can cure disease, but imagery has a long history of healing in shamanic and other native cultures and is recognized as an effective stress management tool by western medicine, often in conjunction with relaxation and meditation. Some studies have shown imagery can boost immunity by increasing defenses, such as T cell and natural killer cell activity in the body. Research also indicates that guided imagery reduces anxiety before surgery and helps cancer patients manage the side effects of chemo more effectively. The following story is one man's experience of the real effects of guided imagery.

"Going Into Orange"

Geoffrey was a young man with lymphoma. He was looking for ways to calm his anxieties and rekindle his interest in life, but nothing much was working. He struggled with meditation and didn't like journaling. He responded to relaxation training in sessions at the hospital, but didn't practice at home. Guided imagery was an instant hit. He pictured himself at a cottage by a lake and immediately felt relaxed. It was autumn and his imagination captured the resplendent color of the trees: yellow, orange and red. As he continued to practice, he found that more and more his focus rested on the orange colored leaves. He called it "Going into orange." One day at a regular appointment, his doctor took his blood pressure and reported it was high. Geoffrey said, "Give me a moment." He closed his eyes, took a deep breath and went "into orange." Before the astonished eyes of the doctor, his blood pressure immediately lowered to the normal range.

Other Benefits

Imagery is a powerful tool because it speaks more directly to the body than words. For example, imagine you are in a doctor's office waiting for test results. Your mind is whirling with all possible outcomes and you tell yourself to relax. Does that work? Not usually because your mind continues to be active. But if you are able to take a deep breath and imagine yourself in a place where you feely truly relaxed, your body responds directly to the image and begins to relax. When your body relaxes, your mind follows suit.

Many people use imagery effectively when they are undergoing stressful or invasive procedures:

I was very scared about taking an experimental drug. My body was clenched and my veins were closed. Two nurses tried unsuccessfully to administer the drug. They went away for ten minutes. I closed my eyes and imagined a warm energy moving through my body. When one of the nurses came back, my body was more relaxed and peaceful. She easily inserted the needle.

I felt anxious about having a Hickman line inserted into my body. I reassured myself that what I was going through was not so bad. I trusted my doctor to do a good job and then I imagined angels in the room. At first I simply said the words to myself, but then I actually felt the presence of angels – I could feel their wings moving. It was very comforting and the procedure went well.

When I was having my PICC line inserted, I imagined riding my horse through nature. I described out loud the movement of my horse, the swish of his tail, and our special communion together and the joyful feeling of being in the woods. Not only did I relax myself, I entranced the entire nursing staff.

Try It

- Close your eyes.

- Take a few deep breaths to relax your body and mind. Relax into your breathing cycle as described in breath awareness and mind/body relaxation. Be open to the experience and easy with yourself.

- Imagine a setting that is deeply peaceful for you. It can be a place you know or a place you make up. It doesn't matter. What matters is that you can picture yourself there with all your senses and feel the powerful effect it has on you.

- Let your worries drift away. Tell yourself that in this moment, you have no anxieties, no concerns, nothing can bother you.

- Picture your setting as vividly as you can. See everything there is to see, hear, smell, feel or touch. For example, if you are at a beach, note the infinite horizon and the different colors of sky, water and sand. Hear the sound of the waves and relax into that comforting rocking rhythm. You might wish to see the sun setting or rising over the water. Take in the sound of the birds, feel the touch of the sand and the gentle warmth of the sun on your skin. Absorb the fresh clean air and savor the salty tang of the sea air.

- Above all feel the powerful relaxing effect this place has for you in your body, mind and spirit. Let go into this peace.

"I Can't Do It. Nothing Happens"

People tell me they can't do guided imagery because they can't see pictures in their minds. Using mental imagery does not take any particular skill; it is something we do naturally all the time. Where are your house or apartment keys right now? How many windows do you have at home? You are using some form of mental imagery to answer those questions. Guided imagery is not necessarily about conjuring pictures. While many people do see vivid pictures in their minds, others do not.

Yes You Can

The key is to use ALL your senses: sight, sound, smell, feel and touch to create images of peace. You don't have to see vivid images to relax. Sometimes it is a sound that has a powerful relaxing effect; sometimes a smell; sometimes a feeling or a touch. Experiment right now. Close your eyes and hear the sound of water lapping gently at the shore or the sound of a water fountain in a beautiful garden; next smell the aroma of cedar in a warm, sun-dappled forest; now conjure the feeling of being surrounded by kindness and care, like a warm blanket of comfort. Finally imagine yourself in a warm shower and feel the touch of the warm water gently soothing your tired neck and shoulder muscles or the gentle touch of a loving hand bringing warmth and comfort to your body. Which of these scenarios worked most effectively for you?

Practice. Practice. Practice.

You can practice imagery anywhere and the more often you do, the more powerful this technique becomes for you. Your imagery session can last anywhere from a few seconds to an hour or more. The imagery can be simple, such as "going into orange" or elaborately detailed and lengthy. Combining guided imagery with deep breathing, relaxation and meditation is especially effective. Integrate imagery of your peaceful place into your daily routine. This simple tool can have profound effects on your wellbeing if you use it regularly.

I've learned to develop an inner peaceful place that I can go to at anytime through meditation and imagery. Whatever happens in the future, I want to count on that space. I no longer dread all the waiting time at the hospital because I see it as an opportunity to practice going to my quiet place. I use an array of images, forests, birds, water. One of my places is a barn. I smell the hay, feel the comforting presence of animals and the deep peace this place has for me.

Further Practice and Study

Notice how your response deepens and opens with time and practice. Feel free to vary your routine and imagery as it feels right for you. There are many excellent guided imagery CDs and books to help you deepen your practice. Martin Rossman's book, *Guided Imagery for Self Healing* is an excellent resource.

5. Journaling

I wouldn't have tried it if it hadn't been for the Healing Journey program. It didn't have much appeal for me. I wasn't expecting much from it. I was surprised.

Journaling calmed me down when I was upset. Nothing else helped.

What is Journaling?

There are many forms of journaling. For our purposes, journaling is writing about your emotions – the thoughts and feelings that get you worked up. These disturbances can be subtle, everyday events that build over time to irritate you, like a family member leaving dirty dishes at the sink, or a thoughtless comment from someone you know, or being cut off in traffic. They can be more challenging – such as feeling unworthy or unloved – health concerns for yourself and your loved ones. Sometimes the disturbances can be overwhelming – a life threatening crisis, loss of employment, divorce or death among close friends and family.

What is NOT Journaling?

We are not talking about a daily record or a diary. They have their place, but that is not what we are focusing on here. We are concentrating on descriptions of thoughts, feelings, and events that disturb your peace of mind.

What's the Point of That?

Won't writing about it get me more upset? Won't I just get worked up all over again? Initially you may relive the emotional charge as you write. You may get "hooked" again by whatever is bothering you. But the process of writing also gives you some space for reflection. This is important. You are not simply rehashing the incident; you are looking for greater understanding of the experience. As you write, you may find unexpected clarity by the simple necessity of translating your mesh of thoughts and feelings into words: an "Aha" moment. Even if there is no clarity forthcoming, the simple act of putting words onto paper forces you to discharge some of the pent up feeling. Many people are surprised by the relief they feel putting words to paper. One woman said it was like taking out her garbage. Just as she cleansed her house of trash once a week, journaling was regularly clearing her body and mind of toxic disturbances.

Ultimately the point of journaling is to develop greater insight into patterns of thinking, feeling and behaving that get in the way of your happiness and peace of mind. With new awareness comes opportunity for making changes in the way you respond. You may not be able to change events, but you can change the way you react to them. You can make changes that move you away from distress toward a calm mind and a warm heart.

It was the anniversary of my mother's death and I felt overwhelmed with grief. Writing about it was the only thing that helped. I started off with my sadness and what I miss most about my mom, the friendship, the nurturing and then at some point I started writing directly to her telling her about how hard it is to accept I will never have my own children, how sad I am for myself, how much I need her now. I was crying as I was writing, but I began to feel lighter – it was like my mother was there inside me. I could almost smell her and feel held in her arms. As I wrote, I felt more and more that my grief is a product of love and it is better to have loved and lost than never to have loved at all. The writing brought me back to what I most loved and although the grief was still there, I began to see and feel that grief, too, is love.

What Are the Benefits?

Writing regularly about emotional events can help us feel happier and healthier. James Pennebaker found that college students who wrote about upsetting events had fewer colds and less visits to doctors than students who wrote about mundane events. Later studies by Smyth and colleagues found that patients living with asthma and rheumatoid arthritis had fewer symptoms when they wrote about emotional events, compared to those who wrote about non-stressful events.

Do I Have to Write About My Cancer?

Not if you don't want to. There is plenty of material in your day-to-day life to work with. You can start by noticing the things that bother you at home, at work and in your social circles. Once you feel more comfortable with writing about your thoughts and feelings, you may find yourself drawn to writing about your cancer.

Try It

- Think back over recent events and choose an incident that disturbed your emotional calm. What happened to upset you?

- Start writing about it. Pretend you are a video camera and you can slow down the action to really examine everything about the disturbance: the circumstances, the "hook" and the thoughts, feelings, and behavior that upset you.
- Have you felt this way before? In what circumstances? Is there a pattern here? Is there anything about the way you responded that you would like to change? Have you noticed how your response feeds into the turmoil you experience? What would your wise self say? Your wise self is that part of you that can step beyond the grasp of being "caught up in it all" and contemplate a broader perspective.

Write Freely

This is key. Write without editing – without worrying about spelling, grammar, or the quality of your writing. It doesn't matter. The point is to get it down honestly. Don't change what you are writing to please an imaginary audience or an outside standard. The audience is you and only you. You can rip it up afterwards if that is what you need to do to allow yourself to write freely. Write openly and honestly without any form of censor.

What If I'm Stuck?

Are you stuck because you can't come up with an emotional disturbance? Or are you stuck because you find it hard to write about it? Some people report feeling calm most of the time and cannot come up with an instance of emotional upset to write about. If you truly experience peace of mind most of the time, then journaling, as we describe it here, has limited benefit for you. You could try a gratitude journal instead, as described in chapter six. However, consistent peace of mind is rare. If no upset immediately comes to mind, perhaps it is because you are looking for a major upset to write about. A minor one, even a slight irritation, can still tell you much about your habitual patterns of response. If you are stuck because you don't know where to begin, imagine telling a trusted friend about your upset. Where would you start? If that doesn't work, start by writing about how you don't know where to begin. What gets in the way? If it seems too confusing, write about that. If it seems too trivial or embarrassing, write about that. Just write and see what emerges.

Practice. Practice. Practice.

You will experience the greatest benefits from journaling if you make a regular habit of writing daily. Choosing a regular time, such as first thing in the morning, helps keep you on track. As you write regularly, you hone your skills of observation and this greater awareness allows you to respond with greater clarity and choice in the heat of the moment as challenges occur in your day-to-day life. Also people who write regularly describe the comfort and relief of having a safe place to express what is most on their mind. The journal becomes like a very good friend who can absorb distress without judgment. Rereading what you have written in earlier times can be comforting and reassuring.

As I write, it becomes clearer to me how I feel. Without my journal, I'd be lost. I like going back over my previous entries. For example, I found I felt exactly the same way at the same point in my chemo treatments. It was reassuring.

When I go back and read what I first wrote, I realize how far I've come. Before there was a lot of anger, disappointment and judging. Now, I'm a different person.

My journal is like a personal friend. When I write I get it all out and then when it is on paper it comes back to me, but in a more loving way. My journal changes my relationship to the things I worry about. I feel lighter afterwards. I'm not carrying so much of a burden.

When I'm in the grip of my fears, I write them down. It helps me get perspective. I also write down anything that helps me – wise things other people say or prayers or jokes or stories.

Further Practice and Study

There are many forms of journaling. If you enjoy writing, you may want to experiment with other formats, such as writing a spiritual journal, or a life story. For further study on journaling and healing, consult James Pennebaker's *Opening Up: The Healing Power of Expressing Emotions* and Louise DeSalvo's *Writing As A Way of Healing.*

Four
The Troubled Heart

My husband asked me to put my wig on when we were home alone together. He doesn't like to see my bald head. I should have said to him, "You're bald. I don't ask you to put on a wig." But I was too tired and too hurt to do anything but comply.

The experience of cancer magnifies heart aches accumulated over a lifetime and generates new ones. So much of our emotional wellbeing is rooted in how we feel about ourselves and how we relate to others. Whatever balance we have found in these domains can be uprooted or at least unsettled by cancer and although it is possible to emerge through the crisis, stronger and more solidly rooted, even happier than before, the process is usually a challenge. Friends, family, partners can fall away or fail to support in some important way. Feelings of sadness, shame, anger or hurt can be complex and confusing. Cancer patients may be uncertain of what to acknowledge and what not to acknowledge, when to protect loved ones and when to be honest and open with them and with themselves. They may not even know how to describe how they're feeling, except that their hearts are aching in some heavy and forlorn way.

Pressures at Home

Cancer is like a rogue wave, appearing unexpectedly on the horizon and then crashing in with full force over patient, family and friends shaking everything up for a while. There are pressures on every front – scheduling multiple medical appointments, processing relevant information and absorbing and disclosing unwelcome news. Patients and their partners need to juggle responsibilities at work and home to accommodate appointments or arrange to take time off. Financial pressures can also mount from loss of work and the many new incidental expenses related to managing illness.

Under such pressure, some couples and families come closer together, others wrench further apart. In support groups there are many stories of both. Whenever a patient describes an ideal scenario of a warm supportive partner and a network of caring friends and family, it is always gratifying to hear. But there are many who do not share these circumstances. Partners, family members, friends can fall short when they are needed the most. Living with cancer means living with the hurt of this experience. Often problems existed before, but grow worse with the pressures of cancer. Here are some examples:

My mother thinks only of herself. When I told her I had cancer, her first response was, "How am I going to get through this?" She had me dead and buried and had her own dress picked out for the funeral.

I practically have to have a nervous breakdown before my husband realizes I need help. I can't do everything myself. He doesn't support me. He just carries on as if nothing has changed..

My husband doesn't like me to look sick. He pretends there's nothing wrong. Once he came home and found me in my housecoat. "What are you doing in that? You should be dressed." He's impatient when I take longer to do things and he never understands that I need to come home early from social events. It's like I'm not allowed to be sick.

My friend went on and on today about her sore knee. I've just learned my cancer has spread and she didn't even ask how I am. All she cared about was her knee.

I phoned my best friend from high school to tell her about my cancer. I haven't heard from her since. Months go by and I hear nothing. Then she sends me a joke email. Does she think this is funny? If she can take the time to send me a joke, couldn't she take the time to say, "I'm thinking of you" or "How are you doing?

The hurts may be large and longstanding – siblings not talking to one another, family members who refuse to acknowledge illness or make any concessions for it, good friends who completely fall away. Or they may be smaller – when people are well intentioned but say hurtful things or lack the capacity to care and support in ways meaningful to the patient.

My sister thinks she is being supportive by asking a lot of questions I can't answer. I guess this is how she hides her own fears.

My friend tries very hard to be supportive but insists I have a benign tumor and blocks any talk of cancer.

Whenever I start to talk about my feelings, my husband jumps in and cuts me off and says, "You're going to be okay." It makes him feel better.

If I ever acknowledge pain, my husband tells me, I should go to the doctor. I'm looking for comfort and reassurance, not "shoulds."

The burden of illness is greater when the people you turn to for support are not there for you. The heart is heavy and troubled – emotions vary and change from anger and resentment to hurt and sadness. In such circumstances, patients feel alone, betrayed, abandoned and disheartened.

Feeling Alone

There is a picture in our Healing Journey archives, drawn by a middle-aged patient named Christine, who felt cut off from family and friends. She drew herself alone in a rocket ship, hurtling through empty space, the earth and all humanity far below. Christine is hugging a TV set for warmth and companionship. I cannot look at this picture without feeling greatly moved. She writes: "I am clutching the TV which supplies the only color in my world. I feel loneliness, but more frustration that I cannot affect the affairs of humanity. I clutch the TV in frustration, but also because it supplies the only warmth and contact with people."

The picture powerfully captures a feeling we have all had at times of feeling alone, cut off, and apart from life that hums and bustles along without us. The loneliness in the picture is striking. Christine writes "I feel awkward, silent, marginal."

When we feel this way, we often respond by isolating ourselves even more. Claudia is another woman who felt alone and cut off, but who courageously reached out when she felt most vulnerable. She had the encouragement and backing of her support group. If you are feeling this way, I hope this book will act as a support group for you and help you to reach out to others too.

When Claudia first came to the group she was thin and ema-
ciated from many rounds of treatment for breast cancer, which
had spread to her lungs and bones. She felt life had dealt her a
nasty turn – just as she had found a job she loved and a group
of friends she enjoyed, everything fell apart with the return of
her cancer. She wanted to continue working but her employer
was not able to accommodate her needs and she found she
couldn't manage a full workload. Friends fell away and Claudia
felt more and more alone and resentful about everyone who had
let her down. So much had been taken from her – once an active
hiker, she now could barely manage a flight of stairs.

*I was full of resentment. It stayed in my body in the pit of
my stomach. I'd rant to myself at home alone. My worse side
came out in frustration and in anger. I felt more and more
hopeless and I couldn't snap out of it.*

*This group was critical for me to get the support that I was
missing. Everyone is kind and encouraging. They helped me
see that my withdrawing had made it harder for my friends to
approach me. They encouraged me to call my friends instead
of waiting for them to call me. I was surprised how quickly
others responded when I moved out of isolation and asked for
help.*

*It's still hard for me to participate socially when I feel
exhausted. I want to go home. But I'm no longer angry or
resentful. I appreciate the support I get. I now start my day
with a prayer of gratitude. It really helps me to feel connected. I'm more able to pick up the phone and talk to my friends.*

Connecting With Others

Connecting with others is important to health and wellbeing
and pivotal to warming the troubled heart. Research indicates
that social support is a key element in recovery across many ill-
nesses including cancer, heart attack and mental illness. We all
benefit from encouragement and kindness. Yet reaching out is
sometimes easier said than done. How can you open up to others when you are hurt by what they say? How can you relate to
others when you feel crippled by your own worries and fears?
Isn't it easier to bottle these feelings up and keep on going? How
can you accept help from family, friends and colleagues when
you are so used to relying only on yourself? And what about
fatigue? Often cancer patients are so tired they don't have the

energy for social engagement. All they want to do is go home and collapse. The last thing they want to do is talk about it.

Cancer, Blame and Shame

There was a time when people did not talk about having cancer. It was considered taboo in polite society so people kept their experience hidden and carried on as best they could. And while those days are thankfully long gone, there are sometimes subtle and not so subtle echoes that deeply impact some patients and contribute to their heavy hearts.

I don't want people to know I have breast cancer. I feel I am too young. When I was first diagnosed, I felt like I had a dirty secret and hid it from people. I didn't want anyone at work to know. I worried they'd see me as less competent. When my husband told an old girlfriend that I was in menopause following chemo, I felt that feeling of shame rising all over again.

Feelings of shame and inadequacy as responses to a cancer diagnosis, are not as uncommon as we might expect in our more enlightened times. More than one patient have described their shock and dismay when friends inferred they must have done something wrong to get sick or asked outright, "What did you do to cause your cancer?"

Being part of a support group helps to place these burdens in perspective. Wise voices prevail and recognize that there is no simple reason to explain why people get cancer and certainly no need to blame oneself for it. Feelings are steered away from guilt, blame and shame toward feelings of empowerment and the solidarity that arises from sharing and acknowledging moments of feeling inadequate and vulnerable.

Still societal pressures exist. Our health-focused culture makes such a virtue of health, vitality and youth that it can seem like a failure to be ill. Living in an environment that constantly reinforces the message that you have done something wrong to get cancer is debilitating and heartbreaking.

Personal Responsibility and Cancer

Many self-help books trumpet the exceptional patient and transformative healing so that patients are left with the impression that curing themselves of illness is their personal responsibility. I will never forget a weary patient speaking out at conference on the psycho-social aspects of cancer – "Isn't it enough that I have the disease without this added belief and burden that I must now cure myself of it?"

Just as there is no need to blame yourself for your cancer, there is no need to take on this personal belief that it is up to you to cure yourself of disease. Such pressure adds unnecessary weight to the hefty load already being carried by the troubled heart. We will return to this subject of taking personal responsibility for curing oneself of illness in chapter seven, when we look at the pressures of living with advanced cancer.

Finding Meaning in Illness

People are generally helped by finding meaning in their illness. This is very different than blaming oneself or believing they did something shameful to cause cancer. For example, many people describe illness as a "wake up call" and respond to the experience as an opportunity to review what's working and what's not working in their lives and to make meaningful changes. They may choose to live in ways that are less stressful, reaffirm what is important to them and to appreciate the simple things in life.

Finding meaning is an important element in warming the troubled heart and will be discussed in the next chapter. For now, we are focused on how feelings of guilt, blame and shame contribute largely to the troubled heart of cancer patients. Finding meaning is one pathway through them. Instead of dwelling on these negative feelings, you can find empowerment and meaning in opportunities for healing and renewal.

Cancer and Feeling Inadequate

On good days, most of these concerns are taken in stride. You wake up feeling you are able to get through your day and ready for the challenges ahead. Your heart and spirit are working with you. But on other days the very real difficulties of illness can seem like too much. You are tired, fed up and discouraged. You feel all too acutely the many ways cancer has impacted your world and thrown a wrench into the smooth running of your life. Tired and discouraged, insecurities rise more quickly. Things you may have taken in stride the day before – hair coming away in the shower, the extra fumbling to find a vein for treatment, an insensitive remark by a family member or colleague – now trouble your spirit. On these days cancer exacts a greater toll – you feel inadequate because you can no longer fulfill your roles at home, at work, at play the way you used to; you believe you are no longer contributing to society and that makes you feel worthless; you feel you have lost your looks and vitality and you no longer know who you are without them; you question your past achievements and doubt future prospects. Your heart is sad and your spirit forlorn.

I used to see myself as a strong person. I could do anything. Cancer has taken that feeling away from me. I now see myself as weak. I feel useless because I can't do the things I used to do.

I'm not a productive member of society. I'm not doing anything. My body is betraying me.

Even those with robust self esteem can have days when all they have lost through illness cuts away at their usual buoyancy and leaves them seriously disheartened.

Disclosure to Others

We have already noted how difficult it is to reach out and talk to others when you are feeling down, tired and vulnerable. But it is precisely at those moments, when it may benefit you the most. Who do you talk to and when? The whole issue of disclosure is complex and personal. Some cancer patients talk to no one or a chosen few; others to anyone who is interested and will listen. Circumstances vary and there may be times when it is hard to know what to acknowledge and what not to acknowledge, when to be open and honest and when to be more reserved and protective. Here are some common perspectives on why some people choose to limit disclosure:

I Don't Want Pity; I Don't Want to be Treated Differently.

Anna came to our program one day with an unusual story – a get well card from a friend had thrown her into a fit of rage. She dropped the card onto the ground and stomped on it! We were all taken aback. Anna rarely showed anger in our group sessions, so what had caused her to respond in this uncharacteristic and dramatic way?

She didn't want pity. That's what had precipitated the scale of her response. As we probed further, we learned that Anna wanted to be seen as herself, not as someone living with cancer. She didn't want to be seen as sick. "I want to feel well, act well and be viewed no differently than before." She felt diminished by the sentiments expressed in the card as if her friend was looking down at her because she had cancer. She was used to being admired for her vitality, her looks, her accomplishments. She didn't want that to change. As discussion ensued, she acknowledged that she sometimes resented the good health of her friends and that the anger she directed at the card, was really anger she was feeling at her own situation and the complex array of emotion around feeling diminished and helpless in face of her cancer.

Others feel the same way:

I like it when people say to me, "You look great" and there's no talk of cancer. I don't want pity. When my mother-in-law had breast cancer, she said everyone treated her as an invalid. She wasn't valued. I don't want that to happen to me.

I don't want to be treated differently. People are compassionate but part of me doesn't want them to be compassionate. I don't like the disease. I don't like being seen as a person with cancer. I am not ashamed of being ill but it is like a weakness.

Arlene used to bolt from her car to her house so neighbours wouldn't have the chance to speak to her:

I don't like it when anyone talks to me about cancer outside of this group. I don't want sympathy or the "poor dear" attitude.

"I Don't Want to Dwell On It; I Want to Get on With My Life."

Keeping busy helps many avoid painful feelings about illness. Why dwell on your situation when you can get on with life? It is a very good strategy at times. Some people are brought up to believe in maintaining "a stiff upper lip." Confiding problems or acknowledging fear is considered a weakness. Strong people "soldier on" without the self-indulgence of strong feeling. But if you continue to maintain a strategy of keeping busy and never talking about your experiences, you are not only likely to burn yourself out, you will also miss opportunities for real connection with the people that care about you.

I don't talk about my illness with my friends. I'm "old school." I've been brought up with the belief that you don't talk about problems. You "get on with it." My friends are like that too.

Most of the time I don't dwell on it. I don't talk about it with my family. I live my life as if I don't have cancer.

I like the idea of choosing not to look or feel like I have cancer. I keep it at a distance.

I Don't Want to be Mollycoddled; I Want to Rely on Myself

Sometimes people feel smothered by unwarranted attention. They don't want to talk about cancer or their symptoms because they don't want to be treated as an invalid. Other people feel very strongly they don't want to burden others with their problems. They prefer to keep their experiences to themselves and to fall back on their own strength and resources when they are in need of them. They may be comfortable giving help to others, but not receiving it. Independence and self-sufficiency are too important. This is perfectly understandable at times. However when you hold on too rigidly to the need for self sufficiency and independence, you isolate yourself from genuine connection with others and the understanding, encouragement, and kindness such connection can bring you.

She checks in with me once an hour. Am I in pain? Am I tired? Do I want anything? It makes me feel like such an invalid. I don't want or need this level of attention.

I've always relied on myself. I thought that made me strong and independent. But now I realize when you don't let others in, you're an island. I don't want to be an island. It's hard for me to ask for help. I'm learning.

I know when I give, I receive. But I was more comfortable being a giver. It's hard to reverse the process and accept help. I have to trust my friends are honest with me about their availability to help.

Friendship is reciprocal. Being a friend means being there in the tough times too. Sometimes I resist being helped. When I first got home from the hospital, a friend offered to drive me to do my weekly shopping. I said, 'No' at first, but she convinced me she really wanted to do this for me. I need to relax and just accept what is offered.

I used to believe it was a sign of weakness to receive help from others, but now I feel that accepting help is part of friendship. When you can accept the give and take of friendship, it becomes deeper and more meaningful.

People Don't Know What to Say

It is hard to reach out to others when there is an awkwardness about what to say. Most people mean well, but their own issues or make-up may leave them at a loss for words. Some people are misguided or insensitive and make hurtful or inappropriate comments:

What did you do to cause your cancer?

Just think positively and you will be fine.

You're so lucky. You have a good cancer.

One woman was told "Oh that's too bad. Now your kids will never be normal." No wonder cancer patients decide to clam up after such encounters.

Friends are pussy footing around. They don't know what to say. Some can't even say, 'How are you? I want to say to them, "I'm still me. You don't need to treat me like a weird specimen."

We often laugh in support groups at some of the things cancer patients hear from their friends or acquaintances. We aren't laughing because they're funny, but because everyone identifies with the ups and downs of feeling connected or disconnected by these conversations and the many joys and pitfalls along the way.

Tell them you have cancer and they tell you the stories of everyone else they know who has cancer. This one lived. This one died. This one went to Africa on a Safari. What are they thinking? I don't want to hear about everyone they know who has ever had cancer. I want them to ask what is it like for me.

"You're My Hero"

Cancer patients hear this often. People find it inspiring to witness a friend or family member living with cancer, sometimes with grace and determination, other times – just making it through the day. While many cancer patients feel encouraged and supported by such remarks, others get tired of hearing: "You're so strong. You're so brave. You're my hero." Here are some of the things they would like to say back:

What choice do I have?

You don't see me on my bad days. It doesn't mean I don't have them.

I'm human. I'm doing the best I can.

A hero is someone who rushes into a burning building to save a baby. I'm not a hero. I'm getting through my day. No more. No less.

I can't tell you how many times I have heard from them, "You are so strong. You will beat this." Sometimes I think I am going nuts, because this is really how I feel, and how I wish it would happen, but sometimes I don't want to hear it, I just want to say to them, "Take your head of the sand. I'm really sick and I want to talk about how sick I am, not about how I am going to get better.

Pressure To Be Upbeat

At the heart of these replies is the wish to give a real response, rather than an upbeat one. Our culture places a lot of emphasis on being positive. While there is no question you feel better when you can reframe troubling thoughts in a more positive light, it is also true that doing this constantly without ever acknowledging the full range of your feelings is only a band-aid response. It is superficial.

There is great value in being upbeat at times – often it is what gets you through the day and makes everyone feel better. But if you maintain a tight hold on the need to always present as positive, no matter what is going on, you are going to wear yourself out and you are going to miss opportunities for more open and honest exchanges with friends, family and the world at large.

Sometimes this pressure to be constantly upbeat comes from within. It is a way of keeping painful feelings at bay and convincing yourself and others that everything is fine.

I ask myself every day, "Do I have my wig on? Do I look the picture of health?" I always try to look well. I don't want to disturb my son. He zeroes in on it.

I was so adamant about being positive that I wasn't letting others in. I wasn't letting my family express sadness.

I had a friend who always made a point of looking her very best and insisting she was fine no matter what her circumstances were. I admired the energy, willpower and the love for her family she displayed. But sometimes this effort came at great cost to herself. She hid her pain and exhaustion in cheerfulness in front of her family. When they left for the day, she collapsed and spent the day in bed. Before they came home, she gathered herself together again and presented her upbeat, 'I am fine' image. When she could no longer maintain this, it was hard for her family to give her the support and care she needed. They truly did not understand how sick she was. It was difficult for everyone to acknowledge openly the real nature of what they were facing, how they felt about it and how they might help and support one another.

The pressure to be upbeat can also come from outside sources, as we have noted. "Just think positively" is a refrain cancer patients hear often. Encouraging upbeat words can be very helpful at times to lift moods and provide reassurance. But sometimes "just think positively" is used by the speaker as an automatic defense against difficult situations and feelings. Instead of helping people, such pap words shut down real communication and leave patients stranded with their troubled thoughts and more alone and isolated than before.

I can never talk about how I'm really feeling to my husband. He only wants to hear positive things.

When the heart is troubled, we often respond by shutting down to the outside world. When we are most in need of kindness and encouragement from others, we are least likely to seek it. We take a guarded and defensive posture to get us through the day. Some people never talk about their illness to anyone.

I never let on when things are difficult for me.

I'm reluctant to admit pain. I tend to be very stoic.

Only place I talk is here . . . no one hears about it. I can't open to others.

When I feel at my lowest, I retreat. Despite my network of friends, I pull back. You can't always be on the up curve; it's not all about triumph.

I have a hard time sharing "I'm really miserable" with others. I retreat. I avoid. I duck phone calls. Maybe I'm not entirely forthcoming. Until I get things under control – until I can get back up again. Then I can face the world.

I Want to Protect the People I Love

Many people keep their situation tightly guarded and their more troubled feelings firmly controlled because they want to protect their family. Naturally it is important to take into account children's ages when making decisions about what to disclose and not to disclose. Young children are helped by being told a parent is sick and everything is being done to help the parent get better. But often the need to protect goes well beyond consideration of ages. Adult children are often kept in the dark because a parent believes it is in their best interests to keep them sheltered from bad news or troubled feelings.

I can't say I'm going to the doctor without the whole family freezing. I hear all the bad news and then go home and tell my daughters everything is fine.

I talk to my kids about my cancer. But I tend to tell them "it's okay" even when it's not. I don't want them to change their lives because I'm sick.

I can't always tell my husband how I'm feeling because he is alarmed. I can feel his stomach knotting. I want to protect him.

My children are in their late twenties. I don't want them to be burdened with thinking of me as sick. I want them to get on with their lives. I don't talk about it but they understand the seriousness. I don't want to force it on them. I deal with it intellectually. Emotionally, I keep it at a distance.

Who is Being Protected?

How much you disclose and to whom depend on your temperament and circumstances. Even if you decide to hide information from others to protect them or to limit intrusion into your life, it is still important to reach out to others for connection. It is also important to be honest with yourself: who is being protected when you adopt this guarded stance? There may be good reasons to keep bad news and difficult circumstances from some loved ones or to limit disclosure of your illness in your working world. But if you are always tightly controlling what is said and not said, perhaps there is more behind this behavior than protectiveness of others or need for privacy and independence. Perhaps you are protecting yourself from your own troubled heart.

Benefits of Being Open

This book is based on the premise that cultivating a warm heart is the most important thing you can do to promote healing. Opening your heart to others is the very fabric of healing change. Laughing and crying with the ones you love expresses caring for one another. Allowing the full range of emotions to be voiced reaffirms your humanity and spirit. It gets at the very essence of what is important in life.

> I believe it is important to take opportunities now to tell loved ones what they mean to us. We don't normally do that in our family. The first time I hugged my mother I was over 50 and she responded like a board. Our family didn't show love for one another; it was just understood it was there. But I changed that. Before she died, I told her what she meant to me. I'm really glad I did.

> When I was first diagnosed I wouldn't talk about my cancer to anyone, not even my husband or kids. I wasn't going to burden anyone – I wanted to handle everything by myself. But resentment started to build up. I was holding everything in. It wasn't good for me. Now I'm not afraid to talk about it anymore. I'm more at peace. The more I share with my family, the more we are sharing together.

When you protect your loved ones from knowing the reality of our situation, you are making judgments about their resources to handle such knowledge. This may be wise with young children, but older children and adults may speculate more is going on than they are being told. Their imaginations may conjure worse scenarios than the ones you are protecting them from.

You also clamp down on your own range of feeling since you need to maintain the appearance that all is well. The pressure of maintaining an "upbeat" front, when you are not genuinely feeling that way is exhausting. You restrict the range of feelings your family and friends are allowed to express. In this atmosphere of "not knowing" everyone must play along with the story line, knowing it is not the complete picture, or being genuinely confused about what is true and not true. When you share more of your experience and how you are genuinely feeling, you create the opportunity to hold these difficult feelings together and for the possibility of a warm-hearted exchange of tenderness, support and encouragement. It lightens your load. You are no longer alone with your troubled heart.

My children ages 31 and 27 both told me in their own ways that they'd be really upset if I hid anything from them. It helps me to know they can deal with it. I don't feel I have to hold anything back. It spreads the pressure. We don't dwell on it. It's not as if we are talking about it all the time. But being open with them helps to keep us feeling close and warm together – that's the feeling – just people together handling this.

I used to be never talk to my family about my cancer. I wanted to protect them. I didn't want to hurt them. But now, with the group's encouragement, I've started talking to them. It is probably the best thing I ever did. It's amazing the support that has come forward. It was so hard to keep it inside me all the time.

Selective Disclosure

Being open doesn't mean you have to wear your heart on your sleeve or constantly dwell on the more challenging parts of illness. There are times for disclosing feelings openly and times for getting on with life.

I have heart to heart talks with my best friends and I can spill out everything. I pick and choose those times. At regular social gatherings, I like to talk normally – not about cancer.

June believes in "walking the line carefully" between open disclosure and protecting her adult daughter. Her daughter knows she has metastatic breast cancer and that there is presently no curative treatment. She tells her daughter she expects to live many years and new experimental treatments come available all the time. She is hopeful something may come up for her. She has cried with her daughter and conveys "that it's okay to feel despair at times. You don't have to be completely stoic." At the same time, she doesn't want to overwhelm her daughter and she encourages her to live her life without worrying about June. She reassures her daughter that she will let her know "if something's going on."

Jessie tells her friends "I'm fine to talk about it" so they can ask questions if they want to. At times she shares her full range of feelings with family and friends, but mostly she concentrates on enjoying her life. She never hides the reality of what she is facing from anyone, but she doesn't "dwell on it" either. "I'm open with people about what's happening because it allows me to be totally who I am." She laughs easily, clearly comfortable with herself and her way of handling things.

Many people choose to withdraw for a while on hearing difficult news. As one woman said, "I have to have some time to myself to figure out my own response before I can talk to anyone else." Others point out the need to be selective about who you talk to as some people don't have the capacity to listen and others simply drain your energy, rather than help restore it.

Acknowledging Vulnerability

Being less guarded means becoming more comfortable with your own situation and allowing people to express their love and care for you without you shutting them down. You don't have to be constantly strong, brave and uncomplaining. Such a stance tends to shut people out. Being more open allows for the joy and intimacy of real connection with others.

Normally I'm a very private person and I don't talk openly to others about my situation. But I find when I'm more open about it, others don't pull back. A cleaner came to the house last week and I told her about my cancer. She responded with such care and compassion. She told me she would pray for me. It made me feel good.

I've learned from this group that the give and take of a relationship rises above anything else; the feeling of being open and connected with others. I've learned to take more risk in letting people get to know me. I feel more grounded.

I'm not trying to put on a brave face all the time anymore. Now I can reach out to others and have others reach out to me.

Talking to others about what I'm going through has light-ened the load. It doesn't get rid of it, but it does share it around. It takes up too much energy to keep up the façade.

Authentic Connection: Magic Wand for the Troubled Heart

The troubled heart hungers for real connection – an authen-tic exchange in which one can talk freely and openly about one's experience and be heard with empathy and understanding and without judgment, advice, or a ready answer. It is the quality of really being present with another. If there is a magic wand for the troubled heart, it is this real exchange – the presence of empathy, care, and connection.

As a facilitator of support groups, I know the very special quality that emerges when there is a feeling of safety and trust in the group. When people feel comfortable and secure to talk openly and honestly about their experiences, the very finest of human spirit emerges. The quality of support is open, warm and accepting. When that fine spirit emerges, the group can hold the full range of experience: stories of things getting better and sto-ries of things getting worse; times of joy and peace and times of despair and stress. The ability to hear and be present radiates through the ups and downs of each story like a healing pulse, so that the weight is lightened and sometimes transformed. One person described this as relating "soul to soul".

I can say things here I can't say anywhere else.

Being part of a group who are so honest is very important to me. Every time someone speaks, I can feel the rawness of what they are saying: there is no attempt to cover that up. I really love that. Truth telling is important. People say things I wouldn't say, yet I can see how helpful it is to that person. That's what is so beautiful about the group – each of us, no matter how open we are, we are just this tiny little speck of what the whole is and so by having six specks say what they think, we get closer to the truth.

The connection I experience in the group is unlike any-thing else. It's as if my fellow group members are as close as brothers and sisters. Really, it's closer because we're talking soul-to-soul when we're in the group.

Reaching Out

Feeling safe to talk openly is key. It is important to reach out to someone who is able to listen in a warm-hearted, non-judgmental way. Often partners or close family members have difficulty listening because naturally they have their own strong feelings about what is happening to you and it may be hard for them to listen in an open accepting way. Or it may be you who wants to protect your partner or family member from your feelings.

Possibly there is no one around who can listen to you in this way. If that's the case, there are many other opportunities for reaching out and getting support. The internet offers a wealth of resources for online support groups and chat rooms. Community resource centres, such as Wellspring, offer an array of services and programs, including support groups.

Hopefully this book too acts as a form of support group – a place to find comfort and resonance from the wide range of voices that speak openly about different experiences. Recognizing your own experience in the voices of others helps you to know you are not alone with your feelings or your situation. When people are asked what they value most about support groups, they reply "No one understands what is like as well as someone going through the same thing" and "It helps to know I'm not alone."

The next chapter focuses on ways to warm the troubled heart. The first part looks at all the factors that get in the way of reaching out to others and describes how to let go of negative feelings, such as anger, shame and hurt. The second part focuses on enriching spirit and opening up to feelings of joy and peace. Remember, wherever you are in your path to a calm mind and warm heart is fine. Whether it is a good day or bad day, there is always the possibility of moving in the direction of warmheartedness.

Five
Warming the Troubled Heart

Love is like a beautiful ball that we toss back and forth. The more we play, the better we get and the better we get, the more we play.

I believe I'm part of something bigger, smarter, happier. I believe our goal in life is to enrich spirit. My challenge is to create bigger spirit.

The words of the Dalai Lama bear repeating again and again: "The single most important thing you can do for healing is to cultivate a warm heart." It is tempting to scoff at such a simple statement or mock its sweet Pollyanna sentiment. All very well to spout, but what does it actually mean? How does such simple sounding guidance have any real substance in face of the complexities of disease and the challenge of living with illness?

Cultivating a warm heart essentially means fostering warm feelings toward oneself and others. It means letting go of anger, hurt, and shame and other patterns of thinking, feeling and behaving that block warm-heartedness and opening up to feelings of joy and peace. It means learning to forgive, accept and trust. It means radiating and receiving love.

Love is the essence of healing. "All you need is love" has become a cultural slogan, popularized by the Beatles song and reinforced by the wisdom of the ages. We discount it nonetheless. It seems too simple an answer and too lofty a goal. Much is lost in its translation into the complexities of day-to-day living.

Perhaps it would help to think of love in a new way – one that translates readily into the context of illness and treatment. No one doubts the power and science of radiation therapy – the use of high energy x-rays, electron beams or radioactive isotopes to kill cancer cells. Radiation affects not only cancer cells, but healthy tissues too so care needs to be taken to limit the area of exposure to these destructive rays. Let's toy with the idea that love is a radiating energy with powerful constructive rays. Giving and receiving love is accessing and moving this potent radiation into body, mind and spirit and outward to the world. It is a constructive force and needs no limits, indeed knows no limits, since once this therapy is accessed, it leaps readily into expansive healing waves.

Granted we are toying with this idea and there is little scientific proof. We are a long way from measuring love scientifically and evaluating its outcome in ways that conform to accepted scientific practices. But it may not be as farfetched as it sounds – new technology is allowing science to understand the relationship between emotions and the workings of the brain. Richard Davidson, a Harvard trained neuroscientist, studied brain activity in Tibetan monks in meditative and non-meditative states using functional magnetic resonance imaging, a recently developed technology that shows changing neural activity in the brain. In meditative states there was a marked shift in the brain's prefrontal cortex from the right hemisphere, which is associated with negative states, such as anxiety, worry and sadness, to the left prefrontal cortex, which is associated with positive states, such as happiness, joy and enthusiasm. Meditating on loving kindness showed the most marked shift in this direction. In other words, radiating love had the most powerful effect. A more recent study suggested meditation influences immune functioning as well. After eight weeks of mindfulness meditation instruction, a group of adult volunteers showed a healthier immune response to flu shots, as measured by greater antibodies in their bloodstream, than a control group of volunteers who did not receive the meditation instruction. After only eight weeks, increases in left-sided neural activity, suggesting greater contentment and happiness, was visible in the meditators, but not the non-meditators.

Other clues that radiating love to oneself and others might bring tangible benefits to mind and body can be found in the work of Dean Ornish, a noted cardiologist and researcher in heart disease. Previously it was thought that heart disease could not be reversed without drugs or surgery, but Ornish's groundbreaking program proved otherwise. His program included a low fat diet, exercise and stress reducing interventions, such as practicing meditation and yoga, joining a support group and opening the heart to forgiveness, altruism and compassion. In his book,

Love and Survival, he argues that love has a direct healing effect on our bodies, promoting stronger immune systems, better cardiovascular functioning and longer life.

Even though this does not amount to scientific evidence for the hypothesis of love as effective radiation therapy, we know it nonetheless. It is not hard for us to accept the idea, it is hard for us to live the idea. We have to move from toying with it as an intellectual idea or hypothesis, to feeling it, living it, making it real for ourselves. This process is made somewhat easier by our own intuitive knowing. Most of us have had experiences, however fleeting, of the power of warm-heartedness. In such moments, sadness, fears and worries drop away and our minds and hearts open to peacefulness and expansiveness.

Stories of such moments abound in support groups – a nurse's caring touch at a moment of anxiety; a stranger's warm smile as they perform some small act of kindness; a young man coming home from treatment, tired, ill and dispirited and having his dog cheer him up by putting his most loved and chewed up dog toy onto his lap. In these moments, we are changed. Something reverberates in our whole being making us feel alive and cared for: a fleeting warm-hearted experience of connection to something larger than ourselves. We know the transformative power of these moments. Here is one such story that stands out:

The most amazing thing happened last January. I was scheduled to go to the hospital for surgery and I was really scared so I contacted the reverend of the United church in our area. We spoke for some time. He made me feel really good. He said to me, "When you are going into the operating room, just say to God, "Lord, I'm in your hands now." I told my mom what the reverend had said and she also felt better.

The day of surgery came and I had to walk down to the operating room at 6:30 am. They don't give sedatives prior to surgery anymore. I was really anxious. My mom, dad and husband were there to see me off. I don't know what I'd do without them. We were walking down the hall to the elevator and I was repeating over and over again, "Lord, I am in your hands now." It was really quiet in the hospital that early in the morning. The elevator door opened and there was a beautiful black woman in the elevator, belting out a gospel song as loud as you can imagine. I can't remember the exact words, but they were something like "The Lord will take care of you and show you the way." My mom and I looked at each other in amaze-

ment and started bawling. She was an angel sent down to make me feel at ease and it worked.

Such encounters can stay with us for the rest of our lives. How do you explain their effect? On the one hand it is simply an unusual story of a woman meeting a gospel singer on the way to surgery. On the other hand it is a life changing moment in which one way of being – mind and body beset with worries and tensions is exchanged for another way of being – mind, body and spirit, warmed and opened by a feeling of being cared for and loved. These moments pass, but the secrets they hold of the transformative power of warm-heartedness stay with us. We can return to these moments when we need a dose of love-radiation therapy. But even more important, we can learn to cultivate a warm heart. As the Dalai Lama says, it is the single most important thing we can do for healing.

Warming the Troubled Heart

This chapter describes the process of warming the troubled heart in two parts: first, letting go of longstanding patterns of thinking, feeling and behaving that block warm-heartedness and second, opening up to feelings of joy and peacefulness through enriching spirit, connecting with others, building community and sharing laughter.

Although letting go and opening up are described separately, they are essentially the same process. As you let go of obstacles to warm-heartedness, you awaken your natural capacity for joyfulness and peace.

Letting Go

How do you foster warm feelings to yourself and to others when cancer brings so many roadblocks? We have already described the many ways the mind and heart are troubled by the experience of illness. Cancer provides a fertile ground for anger, hurt and sadness and these thoughts and feelings are not easily dislodged or reframed. If worried thoughts are like hijackers taking us away from the present moment, then these (anger, hurt and sadness) are the elite terrorists, most capable of wrecking havoc in our body, minds and spirits.

The medical system, as wonderful as it is in providing effective treatment and life saving interventions, is also a source of anger and hurt for some cancer patients and their families. Sometimes cancer is not detected when patients first describe their symptoms. Perhaps the patients are reassured that nothing is wrong, or the symptoms are misdiagnosed or discounted. Whatever the case, these failures understandably rankle and often fester once the diagnosis is clear. What if this mistake cost the patient his or her life? A thought like that takes root and is not shifted or reframed easily.

The medical system can disappoint the patient in many ways – long waiting periods for treatments, scans or appointments; misdiagnosis; failure to fully inform about procedures or possible side effects; preemptive or uncaring encounters with doctors and other health care staff – the list goes on. It is enough that the patient has to cope with cancer, it understandably feels like too much when the patient has to cope with an inefficient or uncaring health system and is forced into a position of advocacy simply to improve his or her chances of getting standard and appropriate treatment and care. It is a refrain I hear in support groups – the effort it takes to advocate for oneself, the dangers of remaining passive, the underlying anger and hurt that it has turned out this way.

Sometimes anger feels good and helps us achieve useful outcomes. It mobilizes us and makes us feel powerful. It makes us determined not to let such a mistake happen again to us or to others. It can lead us to changes that make a difference. But if we stay stuck in the anger, we are not helping anyone, especially not ourselves. When anger continually loops through our minds, it radically narrows our capacity for warm-heartedness. We cut ourselves off from our own peaceful core and we are less likely to receive or give kindness and encouragement to others. The ability to live fully and meaningfully is shut down in the service of this anger.

Holding on to old hurts or feelings of shame is equally unhealthy. Cancer often rekindles longstanding hurts or generates new ones as family or friends fail to be there for the cancer patient in hoped for or expected ways. We have already documented how cancer can make some people feel inadequate at times and the many ways patients can be hurt by the actions or words of friends, family, colleagues or strangers. Feelings of hurt, shame and sadness often precipitate a retreat into oneself, shutting out possible connection with the kindness and care of others. Instead of cultivating warm-heartedness, the hurt person feels only the pain of downheartedness, isolation and sadness. Thoughts associated with hurt feelings lodge deeply into consciousness and are often felt viscerally – a pain in the chest, a stab in the heart, a clench in the belly.

Notice the Hold These Feelings Have on You

The first step in letting go these feelings is to notice the hold they have on you and how they affect your wellbeing. You might take a moment to review the descriptions in chapter two about impact of thoughts on body, mind and spirit. See how it applies to your bitter, hurt and angry feelings. The way people tell their stories of anger and hurt reveal much about their powerful impact:

> I let stuff churn and boil inside.
>
> The anger consumed me.
>
> It hurt like a stab to the heart.
>
> It was eating away at me.
>
> I am torn up inside.
>
> It was a stone on my chest.
>
> Inwardly, I stew.
>
> The remark stung me to the core.

Our words tell us much about the toxic hold these feelings have over us. How do you think your insides are doing when they are being torn, stung, stabbed, churned, eaten, boiled and stewed? Stop and take note. If nothing else persuades you, be persuaded by this, it is in the best interests of your personal health to let go of angry and hurt feelings, no matter how justified they are, or how much wrong has been done to you. Let go of them for your own sake. It is not about excusing or accepting the negligent or hurtful or abusive behavior of others. It is about letting go of the hold these thoughts have over you for the sake of your own health and wellbeing.

What Am I Letting Go Of?

People are always talking about the need to let go of anger and other negative feelings. I don't get it. What am I letting go of? My anger doesn't go away by talking to a friend or writing about it. The thoughts are still there they – continue to tor-

ment me. They still have a hold on me. So what am I letting go of? That's what I want to know.

It's a good question and one that puzzles many. You are letting go of the tight grip negative feelings have over your body, mind and spirit. But letting go is not a one-time event. It is not like dropping a heavy knapsack to the ground and feeling the immediate and lasting release. It is a process. Each effort you take may loosen the grip a little bit. But then it tightens up again. It takes time and repeated effort to experience real effects, but it can happen. It can be done.

Once you are aware of the hold these strong feelings have over you and their negative impact on your health and wellbeing, you make a decision to reduce thoughts, feelings and behaviors that fuel this tight grip and to cultivate a different stance – more open, more accepting, more forgiving.

I'm trying to get beyond fear and anger. I'm trying to be more attune to how my body is reacting and to stand outside myself and be the observer. When I'm angry, my body is tense and charged, and my thoughts are racing. I'm learning my anger doesn't help me. I'm learning not to react so much.

Forgiveness

Fred Luskin leads a research group at Stanford University studying the relationship between forgiveness and health. According to Lushkin, choosing to forgive increases a person's health, happiness, and hopefulness and reduces anger, depression, and stress. Forgiveness means learning to take less personal offense, not blaming others so much and becoming more understanding of situations that lead to feeling hurt and angry. His program encourages people to take responsibility for how they feel and to consider interpersonal hurts in new ways, fostering more positive emotions and less negative ones. Self-forgiveness is also important.

Forgive Yourself

This last point is key. Forgiveness is not only about learning to reduce anger and blame toward others, it is also about learning to be gentler and more accepting of yourself and your own circumstances. Cultivating a warm heart means fostering warm feelings towards oneself as well as others. For many, the hard part is being kind and forgiving to oneself.

I'm feeling more at peace with myself and have forgiven myself for past unhealthy experiences. I used to put myself down for not having a mate or a house of my own. Now I'm more aware of these thoughts when they occur in the moment. I can step back and observe. I'm more peaceful now. Imagery, meditation, and walking have all helped me.

Acknowledge Your Situation

It is important to acknowledge your situation and the cause of your negative feelings. Sometimes it is helpful to write about it as we explored in chapter three on the topic of journaling. To get started, you might try writing a letter to the person who has hurt, offended or failed you in some way. Perhaps that person is yourself. Whatever the case, do not send the letter. This exercise is for you and you alone. The idea is to write freely about the situation and the feelings you have about it. What is most on your mind? What is most important to say? If this person could really listen to your point of view, what do you want them to know about the impact it has had on you. Let the anger, hurt, shame or sadness find its way out of you onto the page.

You have to find it, reach it and then shake it.

This exercise can bring a feeling of immediate release. Writing can discharge some of the tension and stress in your body and bring calm clarity to your mind. Or the opposite might occur – writing about it may steep you once again into angry, hurt or sad feelings. Either way, remember this is a process and moving through these feelings will take time. You might need to write again and again before you feel any sense of release. Remind yourself of your decision to take less personal offense and to look for new ways of understanding the situation.

Strive for Greater Acceptance

Life is messy at times. It doesn't always go the way we want it to or follow the neat script we have laid out for it. A lot of our suffering comes from the fact we hold on tightly to these ideas of the way things "should be" and resist accepting things as they are. As much as we would like to, we can't "fix" other people; we can't make them change into the people we want them to be. We might influence them by modeling the behavior we hope to see in them, but ultimately the only people we can change are ourselves. Instead of replaying over and over the ways someone or something has failed you, try accepting that this is the way things are right now. It may be possible to see this person or these circumstances in a different light. We are all fellow human beings, vulnerable and imperfect at times – circumstances are complex and always changing, despite what we might hope or expect of them. You can learn to be more open and accepting of your own shortcomings and those of others and more at ease with the changes and complexities that life brings you. Instead of feeling angry disappointed, resentful when things or people don't live up to your expectations, or behave the way they "should," you can bring new understanding and compassion to the situation and "go with the flow" more readily. Perhaps you can put yourself in the shoes of the other person and attempt to understand the situation from their perspective. Sometimes you will be surprised at your own revelations:

I let myself get caught in silly games with my mother-in-law. It saps my strength. I don't say anything. I've never been assertive with this woman. I sit there silently and stew. It's not good for me to feel this way. I would like to learn to feel more positively toward her. I would like to reach a place of compassion instead of anger.

I found that much of the anger I was directing at my husband was really unhappiness with myself. I put it onto him, blamed him. It was easier than looking at my own unhappiness. Cancer has helped me see what is and what isn't important. I've let things go. My husband and I are closer now than we've ever been.

I now recognize my anger and catch it earlier. All my unhappiness and frustration with my situation came out as anger at the hospital or it would come out while I was driving. I recognize it now and let it go. I talk to myself. I don't even get angry when I'm driving anymore. Meditation helps to keep me feeling peaceful.

Notice the Benefits:

The person who benefits most from this shift is yourself. As you let go of negative feelings and your resistance to how things are in the present moment, you will find new space to enjoy life as it is. This is the beginning or root of happiness: feelings of contentment and joy naturally awaken. More and more, you will feel at ease with yourself and your world.

Here are two delightful examples of contentment and joy naturally arising after letting go of anger and hurt and practicing forgiveness in one woman's relationship with her mother and her husband. Both stories relate to making jam:

> I went raspberry picking with my Mom for fruit to make jam. I've spent a lot of time examining my relationship with my Mom, remembering and reliving past hurts, analyzing her response to my cancer and experiencing my anger. I went through that with the goal of forgiving, both her and me. This is the first time in memory that I really truly enjoyed spending time with Mom. I was finally willing to forgive, let go of judgment and just accept the two of us where we were at. This means that we can be at different places, yet still be together.

> Lately I have let go of many uncomfortable patterns in my relationship with my husband, such as blaming and criticizing him and wanting him to meet my expectations. In a nutshell I am practicing to be more unconditional in my love.

> I spent all morning making peach almond jam. I was really enjoying the process but then was most perturbed to discover that after ladling the hot mixture into carefully sterilized jars, I had left out the lemon juice. My husband heard my distress and I received such an outpouring of genuine concern and love that I ended up thinking "who the hell cares about the jam"! This kind of scene is becoming a common occurrence at our house – this expression of love. It seems that love is like a beautiful ball that we toss back and forth. The more we play, the better we get and the better we get, the more we play.

Greater acceptance does not mean condoning unkindness or excusing poor behavior. You may or may not choose to reconcile with the person who has hurt or angered you. Sometimes it is unwise to do so, because you might be exposing yourself to being hurt again. In cases where abuse has occurred it is important to keep a safe boundary. However, reconciliation can also bring great joy and healing for both parties. But the choice is yours and what is most important is not the outer act of reconciliation with another, but the inner act of shifting your feelings so that they don't have such a hold on you. Forgiveness is for your health and for your benefit, not for anyone else's.

Catch Yourself and Learn Over and Over Again

In chapter two we described the importance of cultivating an inner observer – the ability to step back and observe your thoughts and thereby break your complete identification with them. This gives you some space to choose to respond differently. In order to effectively shift your thoughts and feelings away from anger, hurt or distress, you need to be able to catch your thoughts and feelings as you think or feel them. Then you can say to yourself, "Stop. There's that same thought or feeling. I'm not going to let this take hold of me right now. I'm going to choose to respond differently."

When you catch yourself, take a deep breath and then use whatever strategies work for you. You might say, "I choose peace. Not this" or "This too, shall pass." Or try any of the techniques described in this book that have brought you peace or comfort, such as practicing relaxation or meditation, imagining yourself in a peaceful place, or filled with healing light. Discharge restless energy by exercising or going for a walk or in any way that works for you. Remember your commitment to loosen and let go of the tight grip these feelings have for you and remind yourself that all this takes time. It is something you learn and relearn over and over again. Trust the process. It takes substantial time and effort to loosen the grip longstanding patterns have on you. You need to catch yourself and learn over and over again.

Each time you go to the edge and back, you learn something from it. It's still painful and hard, but each time gets a little easier because you've done it before. Each time gives you added strength.

Send Yourself Messages: "Easing" . . . "Softening" . . . "Slow Down"

When you are in the grip of strong feeling, you can remind yourself of your intentions to respond differently by using a key phrase, such as "Slow down" or "Just breathe." One woman finds repeating "easing" repeatedly to herself is very effective.

Another likes the word "softening" when she is feeling impatient and critical. Find what works for you.

I tell myself "Slow down" when my thoughts are rushing and I start feeling stressed. Other phrases have been helpful. I find I really like the word "easing." When I repeat it to myself, it calms me.

Letting go of Control, Judgment and Business

There are many other patterns of behavior, besides holding on to hurt and anger that get in the way of experiencing warm-heartedness and peace of mind. Among the most common are: a need for control; a constantly critical mind set; and being busy all the time. People who have strong control needs are often perfectionists imposing high standards on themselves and others. They like to "be right" in discussions and feel most comfortable when they are controlling things. In order to get things done "right," they have to do it themselves.

I used to want to fix everyone else's problems. When something happened at work or at home, my first response was, "Now what am I going to do?" I would take that responsibility on myself. Now I know it's not my problem. I don't have to jump in and fix things. I don't have to be so controlling.

I'm not angry anymore. I can pick and choose when I get involved. For example, I don't get worked up in political discussions with my son anymore. Before I needed to press my opinion and prove I was right. Now, I say what I want to say and then I let it go.

The more we cultivate our inner observer, the more we become aware of the constant stream of critical judgments we make as we go through our day – what people are wearing, how they look, how they act, the traffic going to and from work, and all the ways we find blame and fault in others and in ourselves. Underlying all this is the stressful beat of impatience and rebuke. We make ourselves and others miserable. Imagine what a relief it would be to let this go:

I went through a phase where I thought everyone hated me at work. It was really my own critical stance. I was putting out that energy of dissatisfaction. I was critical of others, but what I really needed to do was look at my own frustrations with myself and my life. Now I'm more accepting of myself and others. It feels good.

The more I practice, the more I consciously stop my mind from criticizing, the more peaceful I feel. I started letting go when I started the process of forgiving my mother. It was like learning a whole new language. I'm getting more comfortable with it now. I'm trusting it more. With trust comes peace.

I am barely ever critical of myself anymore. My core is coming through. I like it.

Another common pattern of behavior is keeping very busy. Sometimes this is a good strategy for a while. It can distract us from disturbing thoughts and feelings, allowing us some time to assimilate what is happening without feeling overwhelmed. But if we are constantly busy, we are not only in danger of wearing ourselves out – we also lose opportunities to slow down and appreciate life and to enjoy warm-hearted connection with others.

I was race, race, racing through life. I never kept my life in balance. My work was always important and everything I did well. I did perfectly. But I didn't know how else to do something: it had to be done perfectly. After getting cancer, a lot of priorities suddenly changed. I had more quality time and heart-to-heart talks with the people I care about. It was probably the first time ever I totally let go. I don't care about being busy and doing things perfectly anymore. I'm more interested in the calm flow of life now and spending time with the people I love.

Letting Go of Fear

Living with fear as a constant companion paralyses us from living. This book began with the topic of fear because cancer begins that way too – as soon as you hear those words, "You have cancer," fear enters your body, mind and spirit. How you manage that fear directly impacts your quality of life. If you repress it, push it away and never face it, the fear lurks deep within and will surface when you relax your busy schedule or in the middle of the night or unexpectedly at times when you were enjoying yourself – at the movies, reading a paper, a family outing.

Facing fears does not mean dwelling on them. It means recognizing the hold they have upon you and using your own resources to summon new perspectives and resources to loosen that tight grip. In chapter one, we described many wise voices on the subject. Writing out your fears often helps to clarify the nature of your worries and to gain fresh perspective.

Writing is a release. It makes fears seem smaller, more manageable. Not such a big deal. It gets you out of that stuck place.

In chapter seven, we return to fear as we address the subject of living with advanced illness. Fear of losing one's life and leaving loved ones, particularly children are the most difficult issues faced by cancer patients and there is no easy way through them. I hesitate to describe these fears in terms of "letting go" for words cannot adequately describe the complicated process of facing these fears and attempting to loosen their hold. However many do find ways of coming to terms with what is happening to them so that they are not held constantly in fear's tight grasp.

It is not only major fears that figure in the "letting go" process: everyday fears and anxieties can cripple you and prevent you from enjoying life – social fears, fears around failure, competency and self-worth. The experience of cancer can acerbate whatever tendencies you have in this area. Sometimes it actually helps by putting common worries and anxieties in perspective. For example, some people think, "If I can deal with cancer, I can deal with anything. I don't need to sweat the small stuff." Letting go of these everyday fears and anxieties is the same process as managing thoughts more effectively and letting go of strong emotions, like anger and hurt: i)developing greater awareness; ii) making different choices; iii) reframing and cultivating new understanding or perspectives: and iv) practicing whatever strategies work best for you.

Opening Up

As you let go, you open up. Just as anxiety, worry and fear drop away in those fleeting moments of warm-hearted connection described at the outset of this chapter, when you let go of negative patterns of thinking, feeling or behaving, you open up to new capacities for warm-heartedness and joy. Opening up is expansive and peaceful, and comes through practicing forgiveness, acceptance and trust. Your spirit opens too. As you let go of whatever has a negative hold on you, you enrich your capacity to live life fully and meaningfully. As one woman put it, "I believe I'm part of something bigger, smarter, happier. I believe our goal in life is to enrich spirit."

Enriching Spirit

If enriching spirit is our goal, we can learn a lot from our pets. Frida, a middle-aged woman with breast cancer, was startled to learn her golden retriever had cancer, shortly after her own diagnosis. After the initial shock and dismay, there was some comfort in the quality of "being there" for one another as they went through cancer treatments together. One day they went out for a walk after receiving their chemo. As they started out, they were both dragging their feet. While Frida's mind and body continued to drag, Frida's dog found a large stick and bounded about joyfully and happily, totally transformed by the pleasures of being outside and playfully prancing with a stick. In those moments, the dog was fully and joyfully itself, without any evidence of tiredness or illness. Watching her dog respond with such joyful spirit to a simple walk outside gave Frida her own moment of warm-hearted connection.

The story instantly hit home in our group session. At its heart is something we all know – we have tremendous capacity to feel alive and joyful no matter what our circumstances are and to find soulful connection with something larger than ourselves, whether it be nature, or meaningful connection with loved ones, (including pets) or some form of spiritual experience. The story also tells us much about living fully in the moment and the healing benefits of playfulness.

As we open up, we have new appreciation and capacity for all of this: for feeling alive and enriched, for meaningful connection with others, for joyfulness and playfulness and for savouring the beauty that surrounds us – in nature, art, literature and music.

What Opens and Enriches Your Spirit?

What experiences do you have that give you feelings of peace, contentment, and connection with something greater than yourself? We ask this question in our Healing Journey Sessions. Here is a typical list of responses:

- Walking in nature
- Gardening

- Meditation and prayer
- Holding a newborn baby
- Dancing
- Walking by the Ocean
- Singing
- Playing
- Finding beauty in everyday things
- Connecting with pets or other animals
- Listening to music
- Being at the cottage
- Giving and receiving love
- Children
- Running
- Helping others
- Beholding sacred space
- Being aware in the moment
- Tender touch
- Belly laugh
- Feeling connected to God or inner spirit

Now take a moment to fully feel the impact these experiences have for you. Perhaps the following list will capture some of your feeling:

- Peaceful
- Energized
- Alive
- Whole
- Healed
- Quiet
- Harmonious
- Oceanic
- Restored
- Safe
- Cared for

- Infused with love
- Attuned and aware
- Warm-hearted

Cultivating a Warm Heart

You know these feelings. You've had these experiences. You enjoy them and then they pass as your day-to-day reality and mind set takes over. Imagine changing this. Imagine being able to live your day in touch with these feelings. Cultivating a warm heart means purposively directing your day to day awareness so that you live your day in a way that reflects and enriches warm-heartedness. This means not only practicing forgiveness, acceptance and trust, but also regularly making time for activities that enrich your spirit and living your day to day moments infused with mindful and warm-hearted awareness.

How much of your day is spent doing things you feel obliged to do and how much is spent nourishing spirit? If you are like most people, the ledger is heavily bound toward obligation and relatively sparse on the nourishing side. Often people think it is selfish to make time for activities that give them pleasure, so they either forego them or do them tempered with guilt. Think of this time for yourself as healing and restorative time, essential for maintaining wellbeing and balance. It is not selfish; it is a vital component of your overall goal to restore your health and vitality. Taking time to nourish spirit is equally important for caregivers as patients. Everyone will be happier and better able to support and care for one another if time is taken to replenish and embrace spirit.

Building Community

The importance of connecting with others for health and wellbeing has been emphasized repeatedly. Hopefully the wide range of voices in this book has provided some support and comfort for you. Living with a calm mind and a warm heart is hard to maintain on your own. Look for groups or opportunities in your community that will support you in this endeavor. Most localities have a wide range of opportunities from meditation or spiritual groups, religious affiliations, cancer support groups, yoga and retreat centres, and so on. If you are in a small town or rural location, you can always start your own group or explore the many on-line Internet opportunities.

The added benefits conferred by being part of a community and having a sense of belonging cannot be overemphasized. People often ask me after a group meditation or relaxation session why the experience is so much stronger when they practice with others compared to on their own. The answer is simple – the group has its own magic. There is a spillover effect so that relaxation and peace builds and spreads like a healing wave around the room.

Giving and receiving help is another way to build community and create healing opportunities. Learning to accept help openly and warmly can be just as transformative an experience as giving compassionate care. In these moments, we touch on what is most important in life and no matter what our circumstances, we mutually benefit from the sharing and lightening of suffering. This is the essence of community, care and belonging and it is powerfully healing.

I feel full of giving. I don't feel so full of cancer anymore.

Finding Beauty in Everyday Things

As capacity for joy awakens, you will likely experience a new or renewed appreciation for the beauty of everyday things – a heightened appreciation of nature, of music, literature and art, of everyday contact with others and new pleasure in everyday experiences. No matter what your circumstances, life in the present moment offers opportunities for the rich expression of joy, generosity and gratitude.

These two stories of random encounters while shopping capture the potential richness of everyday experience:

Last Friday I was touched by the reaction of an elderly lady choosing tomatoes on special. She was looking at a display of mostly soft tired looking tomatoes so I showed her my bag and pointed to the stand where they were. She was so pleased she kissed her hand and touched my face and I was filled with happy warmth – it was lovely.

I was at the dollar store and there was a young girl ahead of me in line. She carefully put four quarters on the counter for her purchase. She had no other money. The checkout girl took the money and said "thank you." The little girl left the store. *Before the checkout person turned to me, she reached under the counter, pulled out her own purse and took out the tax money for the little girl's purchase. I was so moved by her quiet kindness. It made my day.*

Laughing and Playing

I lose a sense of time. Art gives me a chance to play. I am quite controlled otherwise. When I create things with art, I feel like a playful delighted child.

Laughter makes you feel alive.

Contrary to what people expect when they think of cancer groups, we spend a lot of time laughing. At its best, laughter opens us up and connects us together. When we can laugh at ourselves and our situation, we find inner warmth and resourcefulness to handle our circumstances. Laughter feels good and mobilizes our spirit.

Betty was an elderly frail woman living with advanced cancer. She had never married and the little family she had was widely scattered. She had several good friends and liked living alone, except she worried about being on her own as her illness progressed. One day she came to our group with twinkling eyes. "I have a new boyfriend" she announced. "He is tall and black with deep brown eyes and he slept at my side for the last three nights." We were all wide eyed and speechless, eager for more. Betty laughed, clearly enjoying herself. "He also has four legs and a tail." Then we all laughed enjoying the joke with her.

Lisa came to the group carrying a shopping bag. Inside were three wigs, blonde, flaming red and brunette. She playfully modeled each one, taking on different persona each time. Each wig and persona had a different name. She had fun teasing her husband with the different wigs. "Who do you want to date tonight dear? Wild Zelda, sexy Marilyn, or conservative Mary Jane?" Everyone enjoyed this playful handling of a very difficult situation. They knew first-hand the devastating feel of hair falling away and spirit plummeting. They laughed all the more.

Cynthia was puzzled when her daughter asked her for a slice of bread to take to school for show-and-tell. "Why do you want a piece of bread?" she asked her four year old. "Because you have bread cancer" came the matter-of-fact reply. We all enjoyed a good belly laugh over that one.

Humor is possible and rewarding in even the most difficult of circumstances. The chapter on living with advanced illness contains many examples how humor opens spirit and lightens suffering. Norman Cousins wrote a book, *Anatomy of Illness,* in which he chronicled his recovery from a life threatening illness through the use of humor. He believes laughter mobilizes the body's innate healing processes and recommends a steady diet of laughter, jokes and funny movies. Whatever the case, there is no question that sharing laughter enriches spirit and expands and warms the troubled heart.

Moment to Moment Awareness

The real challenge, though, is to live your life in a warm-hearted way that makes a qualitative difference in your daily life: to live moment to moment with a calm mind and a warm heart.

Living the present moment with greater awareness means constantly making choices to let go of strife and open up to peace, time and time again. As the present moment unfolds to the next present moment, you maintain this awareness. When you are in the car and someone cuts you off, when you are in the grocery store in a long line, when you encounter stressful moments at home, the office or out with friends, you catch yourself in the moment and make a choice to move toward peace away from distress. Here are two perspectives on living the present moment with such awareness:

I often use "this is the now" to myself when I am feeling impatient! It helps me focus on what is going on and what the other person is speaking about – and as I tell myself that "this is my life at this moment" whatever the person is saying or doing becomes a lot more interesting and important. It has become a key learning experience for me to become more accepting and tolerant and I am constantly working on becoming less impatient.

My biggest learning is that Now is not today. Now is feeling, touching awareness. It is not Now until you focus on it. You bring full awareness to what you are thinking, feeling or doing.

Daily Practice and Ritual

Developing a daily routine that reinforces peacefulness and warm-heartedness is helpful in building and maintaining this awareness throughout the day. Whether it be daily meditation, journaling, imagery or some other technique, steady adherence to your practice is one of the surest ways to foster stable and lasting peacefulness. In the following chapter, five new techniques are introduced to help you sustain warm-heartedness.

Daily rituals are also an effective way of making real your intention to live with a calm mind and a warm heart. By bringing mindful and warmhearted awareness to something you already do every day, you begin to live and feel this awareness more and more as you go through your day. The Muslim call to prayer five times a day is a wonderful example of how ritual can work to "reset" one's bearings toward peacefulness away from the hubbub of daily life. We can do this too by finding consistent and repetitive ways of affirming and resetting our intentions in our everyday activities. I was surprised and delighted by one woman's description of making a ritual of her morning cup of coffee. She savored every part of making the coffee, the smells, the sounds, the motions. She used the same slow deliberate process each morning bringing her full attention to each step so that it had a peaceful, fluid, meditative feel. She gave thanks along the way for the beauty and smell of the coffee bean, the growers, the pickers, and all the handlers who brought this luxury to her. The cup, a gift from a friend generated warm appreciation of friendship. No matter what the weather, she took her coffee to her outside deck for her first sip. Her back deck was a peaceful refuge. She loved nature in all its varieties and seasons and stopped to fully appreciate the present beauty before she took her first sip. Then the Ahhhh moment as everything came together in the first rich taste: the extraordinary flavor, the tranquility of nature around her, and her resolve to live her day with peace and kindness. As she described her ritual, every one of us in the group felt her AHHH moment. That is the point. Ritual catches and focuses awareness. Feelings spread out into the day and in our case, to our entire group.

Making morning coffee into a ritual is a good example of how even the most mundane of our activities offer opportunities for resetting our awareness to fully live the present moment and affirm our intentions to live peacefully with a warm heart. Others use the morning shower, a walk to work, grace before meals, greetings and connections with others, the list goes on. A jogger I know stops at a certain bridge on her running route for a quiet moment of reflection and prayer. Some start the day with a specific ritual of asserting an intention, like living the day with kindness and then end the day with a review of how the intention played out.

I particularly like the practice of setting myself something to remember to do for the whole day, especially when I am busy and trying to get a lot done. I ask myself: "What is important? What do I need to remember today?"and I remind myself, if I can't change things, to be more accepting.

For most of us, living your life with this moment to moment awareness is something you build toward rather than achieve. You are moving toward peace, away from distress. That is all you need to keep in your mind and heart. Wherever you are in this process is just fine. No matter what your circumstances are or how many challenges you face within yourself or from others, there is always the possibility of taking a small step toward peacefulness, away from distress. Little by little, step by step, this intention toward a calm mind and a warm heart can make a significant difference no matter where you find yourself in this moment.

Six

Five Techniques to Open and Warm your Heart

1. Garden Gate

2. Loving Kindness Meditation

3. Gratitude Journal

4. Inner Healer

5. Healing Light

These techniques build upon the skills you learned in chapter three on breathing, relaxation, meditation, guided imagery and journaling. Breath is the centrepiece – the bridge to relaxation and deep inner peace. As you hone your skills in breath awareness and meditation, you learn to release tension, focus your mind and open into new expansiveness and peace. As you practice relaxation, you become more aware of how tension feels in your body and the places where you typically hold it; you learn the warm, open feeling of relaxation and how mind and spirit synchronize with a relaxed body, bringing peace and comfort to all levels of your being. Meditation and journaling present opportunities to cultivate your inner observer and to recognize more readily patterns of thinking, feeling and behaving that lead you to distress. Through guided imagery, you experience first-hand the power of your imagination to mobilize healing energy and foster peacefulness.

Challenges to Practice

These skills are the basis for achieving inner peace and contentment no matter what your circumstances. The challenge is to stick to them long enough to appreciate their benefits. Once you know first-hand that they can change how you think, feel and behave in times of stress, then you know you have a powerful set of tools at your disposal. The more you practice, the more peaceful awareness becomes part of who you are and how you live your life.

However you have to maintain your practice in order to continue to receive the benefits. Wouldn't it be wonderful if we had a "reset" button which we could press at times of stress and instantly reset our mind, body and spirit to peaceful channels, but it doesn't work that way. Just as maintaining physical fitness requires regular exercise, maintaining peaceful awareness requires regular practice. The good news is once you know the benefits, it is easier to build upon and recover these feelings, even if you take a long break from practice. At some level, you know the inner peacefulness at your core, even if you can't always access it when you need to. Knowing it is there, can give you some light when you experience moments of darkness.

Review of "Making it Real"

We discussed in chapter three the importance of meaningful experience – how you feel, live and personalize your practice so that you "make it real" to yourself. Such experiences have a "feel right" – quality and help to reinforce and deepen practice. "Making it real" is the process by which you integrate meaningful experience from your practice into your day-to-day life and vice-versa. Here is an example of a woman "making it real":

> About three months ago I created a meditation room based on the room I pictured during a guided imagery exercise. The color of this imagined room seemed important and I was able to recreate the exact color in the paint. I have a small table on which I place objects of meaning including my animal guide from the Inner Healer exercise and candles and incense. This room is powerfully relaxing for me – within seconds of sitting down to meditate, my palms tingle and the muscles in my face soften and tingle. As meditation continues, balls of energy accumulate in the palms of my hands and seem to pulse and roll around.

Perhaps there is an image or phrase that helps you to relax more deeply which you can use to enhance your practice or as a cue in your daily life to remind you of peaceful awareness. I like the following example because it is counter-intuitive. Who would have thought saying to yourself, "Life's a bitch and then you die" would bring comfort? But it did just that for one woman, who always brought a unique blend of humor, wisdom and common sense to our group sessions.

When I learned I had cancer six years ago, I had difficulty thinking clearly and the mantra "life's a bitch and then you die" would sing-song in my mind. This mantra has stayed with me over the past six years oddly giving me comfort. It just seemed to make light of any difficulty I experienced at any given time. I feel we are but sparkles in time, some lasting a tiny bit longer than others. I've reconciled myself to the fact that my time may not be as long as the next person's and it doesn't matter. I feel longevity is not key to living for me nowadays. I look to the essence of experiences and try to appreciate and feel the awe of it all.

The possibilities for "making it real" are endless – it is simply a matter of paying attention to "feel right" experiences and intentionally working with them to deepen your experience and to integrate peaceful awareness into your everyday life.

Opening and Warming Your Heart

As you open up more, you have greater capacity for seeing and appreciating beauty around you in everyday landscapes and experiences. Your heart opens and warms to the pulse of life and the wonder of being alive. Joy naturally arises. The following techniques support the opening and warming of your spirit. The Garden Gate, Healing Light and Inner Healer are all guided imagery exercises to foster openness, forgiveness, healing and intuitive wisdom. The Loving Kindness Meditation and Gratitude Journal develop compassion, thankfulness and warm-hearted feelings for oneself and all humanity.

Each of these techniques can also be used to enhance your practice in breath awareness, relaxation, meditation, guided imagery and journaling.

1. Garden Gate
What Is It?

The garden gate technique is a guided imagery exercise in forgiveness. You imagine yourself in a beautiful garden enjoying the quiet and beauty of nature. Someone you resent approaches the garden gate. You can let the person in or keep them at the gate. Whatever the case, you reflect on your feelings toward this person with a view to softening the hardness, hurt or resentment you feel inside.

How Can It Help Me?

Holding on to resentment narrows our capacity for warmheartedness, for joy and happiness. We cut ourselves off from our own peaceful core and we miss opportunities for exchanging kindness and encouragement with others. In short, holding on to anger and resentment shuts us down. This exercise is intended to help you loosen the grip such feelings have over you and to encourage greater ease, acceptance and understanding of your situation.

What If I Don't Want to Forgive This Person?

That's fine. This exercise is not about excusing the hurtful, inappropriate or abusive behavior of others. It is about changing how you feel inside. Sometimes reconciliation brings great benefit to both parties; sometimes it is best to keep your distance. You control the garden gate. You can let the person in or keep them at a safe distance. Remember, forgiveness is primarily for your health and your benefit, not for anyone else's. However, the exercise does require you to step out of your long held stance and look for ways of opening and softening your perspective. Instead of rehashing the ways someone has failed you, seek greater understanding and compassion for yourself and this person. Perhaps you can put yourself in their shoes and contemplate the situation from their perspective.

Often it is better to start with someone who represents a small resentment or hurt. That way you can gradually work your way up to dealing with the larger, more deeply held resentments.

Create a Healing Space

The garden is a healing sanctuary. This exercise works best if you are deeply relaxed. Conjure a safe and tranquil place. Make it as real and vivid as possible. Nothing can harm you in this special sanctuary. Give yourself permission to let go all your worries in this moment. Like the garden, you are cultivating the conditions for growth and change, planting the seeds for optimal wellbeing and weeding out the stubborn roots of anger and hurt.

Try It

- Loosen any tight clothing, turn off phones and free yourself from other distractions. Create an inner space for relaxation to occur – be open to the experience and easy with yourself.

- Relax and/or meditate. Bring awareness to your breath, breathing in and out slowly, deeply and comfortably. Practice deep inner relaxation, moving through your body, relaxing muscles as you go. Imagine a warm healing energy bringing comfort and healing to your entire body, every part of you relaxing, easing and softening.

- Picture yourself seated on a comfortable chair or bench in a beautiful garden – a place of wonder, mystery, and healing. All around you are flowers in an array of colors: blues and violets, reds, yellows and golds. There is every imaginable color, vivid in the light, shining, as if lit from within. Smell the different fragrances and the pleasing musty smell of earth. Hear the sounds – the buzzing of insects, birdsong in nearby trees, rustling of leaves, the tinkling sound of a water fountain nearby. Feel the warm touch of sunlight and the hint of a breeze on your skin. Imagine feeling really well in this garden. Your breath is rising and falling as a wave of pure peaceful energy flows through you, bringing peace, comfort and healing. Feel the stillness.

- Imagine a gate leading into this garden. Someone you resent is approaching. This person asks to come into the garden. You can either invite the person in or keep him or her at the gate. It's up to you.

- Notice the emotions in yourself. What are you feeling as the person moves toward you or remains waiting at the gate. What is going through your mind? If you allow the person to come closer, have a good look at him or her. Try to see this person in a new light. Why do they behave the way they do? Try to see this person as fallible, like most of us, struggling in his or her way.

- Perhaps you can get up from your seat. It depends on what you're feeling. Maybe you can shake hands or reach out to this person in some way. Perhaps you have an important message to communicate. It's up to you. You may like to return to the bench and sit together and talk for a while. If it's appropriate, you might say "I forgive you."

- Try to encourage a warm-hearted feeling. That's what this exercise is about. Imagine a healing light filling you and reaching out to this other person. Imagine wishing this other person well despite your past history together. Feel the warmth and openness of your healing thoughts embracing you both.

- Now gently bring this exercise to an end. You may want to say goodbye to this person and to see him or her through the gate. Take a moment to notice any change or opening of feeling in yourself. Sit quietly for a few minutes in this healing sanctuary before returning to your day.

Practice. Practice. Practice.

Forgiveness takes time. Don't be disappointed if nothing much happens the first time you do this exercise. Remember, you are watering the seeds and cultivating the ground for new experiences. Perhaps each time you do the exercise you will feel a little more softening and opening inside as you find new acceptance or compassion for yourself, the other person and your situation. Again, it is not about excusing reprehensible behavior, it is about letting go of the hold it has over you and finding compassion and warmth within yourself for life as it is, rather than as it "should" be.

I don't like my mother-in-law. She is self absorbed, opportunistic, manipulative and doesn't care about anyone other than herself. I allow myself to get caught up in her games, never saying how I feel. When I did the garden gate exercise, I did not let her into the garden. I kept her at the gate. She stood there criticizing the garden. She wanted to fix it. I got angry, but didn't say anything. That's how it is in real life. I tried to soften my perspective and reach for new understanding, but nothing much happened except that now I realize that it is not helping me to hold onto these feelings. I'm stewing inside. I do want to change. I would like to reach a place of compassion. I'm going to work at this for my own sake. It helps to hear other people have worked through similar feelings.

When I did the garden gate exercise, I started off with a guy I knew from work. But my father kept appearing instead. This surprised me because I thought I had dealt with my anger toward my father long ago. He's dead now and I thought that chapter in my life was closed. So I asked my father why he was here and that started the whole process of dealing with my unfinished business with him. It took some time, but in the end I felt lighter and more accepting of what happened between us. It opened me up in new ways and was probably the most healing thing I did.

Further Practice and Study

All the established religions and spiritual traditions extol the value of forgiveness for healing. Health care professionals are increasingly focusing attention on forgiveness and health. For example, Fred Lushkin's "Forgive for Good"; www. learningtoforgive.com. See also Daniel Goleman's *Destructive Emotions* for more on overcoming anger, hurt, and other strong feelings.

2. Loving Kindness Meditation

What Is It?

Loving Kindness Meditation is an exercise that focuses on cultivating compassion for yourself and others. First you open your heart to radiate warmth and kindness to yourself, then to loved ones and then to more and more groups until you are directing warm-hearted feelings toward all living beings. For some, the hardest part is directing love toward oneself:

I've been working with a loving kindness meditation, which allows me to be loving and kind to myself – to incorporate the feelings I may have for other people and in other circumstances and finding that within myself, I have been able to be much kinder to myself.

How Can It Help Me?

Chapter five described the transformative power of warm-hearted connection with others and mentioned the work of Richard Davidson on the power of meditation to generate positive emotional states. When kindness and compassion are cultivated, worries and anxieties diminish, replaced by an expansive feeling of warm connection and joy. We have all had these moments, even if they are rare and fleeting. By practicing loving kindness meditations you are intentionally fostering this state of warm-hearted openness and kindness. As your practice continues, you make this more and more a part of who you are and how you live your life. Joy naturally arises in you and extends outward into your world. It can transform your whole being.

"Making It Real"

This meditation involves repeating phrases to yourself to open and warm your heart. For this to have most effect, it is important to really engage your imagination in a personally meaningful way – to really feel the words as you repeat them to yourself, not just mouth them to yourself. If appropriate, change the words so they "feel right" for you.

Try It

- Loosen any tight clothing, turn off phones and free yourself from other distractions. Give yourself permission to take this time for meditation without interruptions, worries and doubts. Free your mind of any plans or preoccupations – be open to the experience and let your mind be at ease.

- Bring awareness to your breath, breathing in and out slowly, deeply and comfortably. Scan your body for any tension, relaxing muscles as you go. Imagine a warm healing energy washing through your body and every part of you relaxing, easing and softening.

- Picture someone in your life who loves you or loved you unconditionally. This person may be living or dead. You might like to picture yourself as a young child or as you are now, surrounded in warmth and loving kindness. If there is no such person in your life, perhaps you can imagine being loved in this way. Conjure up such a person in your own mind or use a religious or spiritual figure that feels right for you. Feel the love and kindness as much as you can. Feel it rather than think it.

- Allow your whole body to bask in these feelings. This love comes to you just as you are. There is nothing you need to do except open yourself to it. This loving kindness comes to you fully and freely without conditions. Even if you feel you don't deserve it, it doesn't matter. The love comes anyway. Let it wash over you bringing you warmth, comfort and joy.

- As you experience this love, repeat these phrases quietly to yourself:

  May I be filled with loving kindness.

  May I be well.

  May I be at peace, at ease with myself.

  May I be happy.

- Let feelings and images arise with the words. Repeat the phrases again and again, letting the feelings of warmth and kindness permeate your body, mind and spirit. Find the images and feelings that best open your heart.

- When you feel the loving kindness filling your own heart centre, you can begin to radiate this feeling outward. Direct this feeling to someone you love. Picture them as vividly as you can and recite the same phrases using their name.

  May they be filled with loving kindness.

  May they be well.

  May they be at peace, at ease with themselves.

  May they be happy.

- After this, you can gradually begin to include others: loved ones, friends, community members, neighbors, people everywhere, animals, the whole earth and all beings. As you practice, you can even learn to extend love toward people who have caused you anger or pain.

- Your session can be as long as you wish. When you are ready, bring yourself gently back and spend a few moments in quiet reflection before going about your day.

Practice. Practice. Practice.

As you continue in your practice, you will find warm-hearted feelings extend beyond your meditation session into your day. Situations that once caused anger, hurt, and impatience, now evoke softer, kinder and more generous feelings. With consistent practice, you emanate warm-heartedness in everything you do, seeing beauty in everyday things and experiences and living life with joy and purpose.

In times of pain, darkness or struggle, you can turn to this loving kindness meditation for inner comfort and warmth.

I woke up in the middle of the night very anxious and fearful about my future. Thoughts and worries kept going around in my head and I couldn't sleep. Then I tried a loving kindness meditation. I imagined the people I love most, each in turn and repeated the phrases about them being filled with loving kindness, being well, happy and at peace. I pictured them in a beautiful healing light. It settled me right down and I went back to sleep. Now whenever I'm really upset or in pain, I turn to this loving kindness meditation. It's the only thing that works for me.

Further Practice and Study

Any book by the Dalai Lama is essentially about cultivating compassion and how this can transform your life. His best seller, *The Art of Happiness* is a good place to start. Karen Armstrong, the noted Oxford scholar contends that compassion is the centerpiece of all religious and spiritual traditions. Her latest book is *Twelve Steps to a Compassionate Life*. Jack Kornfield's *A Path with Heart* describes the loving kindness meditation in greater detail and offers guidance on developing a spiritual life.

3. Gratitude Journal

What Is It?

The gratitude journal focuses your attention on appreciation of all aspects of life. It is a daily practice of noticing, cultivating, and recording moments of gratitude.

How Can This Help Me?

So often we focus on the things we don't like about ourselves, about others, and about our life. We focus on what isn't going well and fail to appreciate what is going well. Resentment shuts us down to the beauty in us and around us. Just as resentment shuts us down, gratitude opens us up. Gratitude and compassion are the antidotes to anger, hurt and resentment. You can't be angry and grateful at the same time. Cultivating gratitude, along with compassion, is the surest way to achieve a calm mind and warm heart, no matter what your circumstances. No matter how awful you are feeling, no matter what the future holds, stopping to notice a moment of kindness or something beautiful can instantly lighten your load. By consciously cultivating this appreciation on a daily basis, this capacity grows and spreads infusing your spirit and your life with joy and meaning.

What If I Have Nothing to Be Grateful For?

Some days can seem like that. Nothing appears to go your way – days when you have received bad news, or are in pain, or feel disappointed and abandoned by the people you need to rely on. Yet those are precisely the days when cultivating gratitude can make a difference by lightening your load and shifting your perspective. Recall the case of Claudia in chapter four, who felt cut off from her friends, and overwhelmed by the relentless debilitating symptoms of disease. She ranted against the unfairness of it all, retreated from the world and spent many days in bed crying with the hopelessness of it all. She continued to come to our group sessions and found relief and support by describing her physical and emotional pain to others. She felt grateful to the group and with their encouragement began a daily practice of starting the day with a gratitude prayer. This small act turned her around making it possible for her to pick up the phone and call her friends instead of waiting for them to call. She was surprised by the outpouring of warmth she received.

There is always something to be grateful for, even if it a very small gesture like the smile of a stranger or the comfort of a blanket, or a warm sunny day. If it is one of those days when nothing seems to warrant appreciation, perhaps you can take some comfort that the day will pass and the next one may well be better. Reciting the mantrum – "This too shall pass. This too shall pass," may help to get you through the day.

Try It

- Buy a blank notebook or journal and keep it in the same place, at bedside or some other appropriate location, with a pen nearby. Dedicate a set time each day to write for 20 minutes. Just before bedtime or first thing in the morning, are good times, but any time that works for you is fine.

- Think back over the past day and write about five things you're grateful for, however big or small. The possibilities are infinite – sun coming in the window, a stranger's smile, feeling well, laughing with a friend, a family member doing a chore, a blue sky, cheerful welcome from a pet, moments of love, kindness and friendship with others.

• Write freely. Do not worry about grammar, spelling or how well you are writing. It doesn't matter. The point is to freely express your appreciation of the good things in your day. Allow feelings of gratitude to well up in you. Enjoy the experience. Truly appreciate these blessings.

• As you move through your day, make mental notes of appreciation. Open you heart and mind to expect good things to happen and notice how they do. Write about that as well.

• Write five things every day. As your gratitude deepens and becomes more automatic, you can shine this new appreciation on troubled areas – relationships with difficult people in your life or dissatisfaction with yourself and your situation. For example, instead of focusing on all the ways an individual annoys you, make a point of finding five things you like about the person.

• Personalize your gratitude journal in any way that feels right for you. Add pictures, newspaper clippings, magazine photos, prayers or poems.

• When you need to revive your spirit, turn to your gratitude journal for inspiration and spirit.

Practice. Practice. Practice.

Any time you stop to appreciate your life more fully will warm and open your heart momentarily. Writing daily about this appreciation and maintaining the practice over an extended period of time can change who you are and how you live your life, bringing lasting joy and peacefulness.

I will always be grateful to the nurse who held my hand when I got the news so abruptly. I want to go back and thank her when I feel strong enough.

I go through my day and make snapshots in my head of people, places and things I'm thankful for. At night I review them; there are always many. When I'm upset I turn to these "snapshots" and they give me such comfort.

I call my journal, "Make Everyday Count." Instead of letting days drift by mindlessly, I make a point of really noticing what I enjoy and writing about that.

Further Study and Practice

There are many other ways to develop appreciation, gratitude, and a sense of meaning and purpose in life. For example you might start a spiritual journal in which you reflect upon what inspires you, what values are most important to you and how you might live your life in a way that reflects those values. You could include inspirational passages or quotes, poetry and anything else that assists you in your exploration of your own spirit and purpose.

Another exercise is to reflect back on the past week, then the past month, the past year, the past decade and so on, recalling good things, joyful moments and all the ways you experienced love, kindness or support from others. For more exercises and practice with gratitude, see Tal Ben-Shahar's *Even Happier: A Gratitude Journal for Daily Joy and Lasting Fulfillment.*

4. Inner Healer exercise

What Is it?

The inner healer is an imagery exercise in which you consult with a wise loving person for guidance and healing. For some, it is a spiritual exercise inviting contact with divine wisdom; for others it is a way of connecting with one's own wise intuition. You imagine walking into a beautiful forest and meeting an animal guide. This animal guide takes you deeper into the forest until you reach the place where your inner healer lives. You meet with him or her and benefit from the words or presence of this wise, loving healer.

What Is the Point of That?

The point is to make contact with an inner voice or "knowing" that bypasses your busy mind. Have you ever had a "knowing" about something that can't be explained rationally? For some people this is a fairly common occurrence – for others, less so. There are many ways this presents – for example you may "know" when you are not being told the truth – or you "know" something is going to happen before it does; you may have an immediate feeling of heaviness or lightness walking into a new place; you may make a decision based on "gut feel" rather than reason; you may find an answer to a problem you have long struggled with "out of the blue" when you are not thinking about it. All these instances are examples of intuition. The inner healer is a way of contacting this intuition for guidance, support and healing.

Who Is This Inner Healer?

The inner healer can be any wise-loving figure. It can be someone you know, such as a loving grandparent or a spiritual figure, such as Buddha, the Virgin Mary, Jesus, an angel, the voice of God, a sphere of light, or have no form at all except as a warm loving presence.

How Can I Believe in This Wisdom? Aren't I Just Making It Up?

There's a difference between contriving an image with your active mind and letting one arise from your imagination when your body and mind are relaxed and at peace. Initial relaxation is a key part of the exercise. At first, it may feel contrived or forced. The more you practice, the more comfortable you will become with the format. You will know when the experience is coming from a deeper place because it will resonate in a meaningful way. There will be a "feel right" quality to the experience.

But if you feel you are just making it up, that's okay too. In his seminal book on "Guided Imagery for Self Healing" Martin Rossman advises you to "Fake it 'til you make it". If it feels forced and contrived, just go along with it. Continue your practice and with time and experience you will be able to distinguish between images that feel like they come from your busy directive mind and images that come from a deeper place.

What If My Inner Healer is Harsh and Critical?

Then it is not your Inner Healer. You have met an inner critic instead. This is an important point. Your Inner Healer is always warm and loving and has only your best interests in mind. If other voices or presences show up, tell them they are unwelcome and send them away.

Create a Healing Space

This exercise works best when you are deeply relaxed. Practice one of the relaxation techniques you learned in chapter three before starting this guided imagery. Adopt an easy and accepting manner, open to whatever the experience brings. Make the experience 'real' for yourself by engaging all your senses in creating a safe healing place where you feel relaxed and at peace.

Try It

- Loosen any tight clothing, turn off phones and free yourself from other distractions. Give yourself permission to take this time for relaxation without interruptions, worries and doubts.

- Close your eyes. Bring awareness to your breath, breathing in and out slowly, deeply and comfortably. Practice deep inner relaxation, moving through your body, relaxing muscles as you go. Imagine a warm healing energy bringing comfort and healing to your entire body, every part of you relaxing, easing and softening.

- Imagine yourself in a lovely country setting on a beautiful day. You are surrounded by grass, shrubs, wildflowers. Ahead of you is a forest. Notice the blue sky, the feel of sunlight on your skin, the sounds of birds and the rustling of leaves. Use any imagery that is personally meaningfull for you. Imagine yourself feeling really wonderful.

- Now picture yourself on a path moving toward the woods. Enjoy the feel of the ground beneath your feet as you walk along into the forest. It's slightly cooler inside the wood; the sun shining in beams of light through the branches, illuminating the path. It is very peaceful and quiet. You feel safe here, any tension you were carrying, now dropping away.

- Continue along the forest path until you reach a clearing. There's a log there and you sit quietly for a while taking in the peacefulness. Now imagine an animal guide is going to appear to take you to your inner healer. Wait a moment or two for this animal to appear. Whatever appears is just fine. Let the animal guide come up to you, greet you in its own manner. You may want to touch the animal or connect with it in some way.

- Follow the animal as it leads you deeper into the forest. With each step you take, you feel you are moving closer and closer to a special healing space. Eventually you reach another clearing, filled with a beautiful light. There is a hut, or a cave with a door, which you are drawn towards. This is the dwelling of your inner healer.

- You can knock on the door, call out quietly, or make your presence known in any way you like. The door will slowly open and your inner healer comes out to greet you. Your inner healer may appear as someone you know, a wise person, a spiritual figure, a being of light or no being at all — just a wise loving presence that you can consult.

- Feel the warmth and wisdom of this being wash over you. Greet your inner healer in any way that feels right for you. There may be something you have come to say or ask. You can bring up any question or concern; or confide something you haven't been able to say to anyone else. Then wait in silence for any answers or messages. These may come as words, or feelings, or in any way at all. Perhaps no answers come this time and that's fine too. Enjoy the warmth and peacefulness of the encounter.

- When you're ready, take your leave knowing you can come back anytime. You will know how to say goodbye and express your appreciation. Your animal guide is waiting for you to take you back through the forest to the original clearing. You wind your way back together in quiet and peaceful reflection enjoying the sounds and smells of the forest.

- You say goodbye to your animal guide, expressing your affection for it and knowing it too will be waiting for you when you return. Sit quietly for a few moments enjoying the comfort and peacefulness of your experience before opening your eyes and returning to your day.

Practice. Practice. Practice.

The more you use this exercise, the more it becomes an effective tool to access inner warmth, guidance, and tranquility. Using peaceful background music may enhance the experience.

I meditate in my special place at least twice a day. I take long walks into the woods and my special healer meets me.

This has been a wonderful new experience. It feels like I'm in a place where the cancer cannot grow. My Inner Healer has helped me remove some of my fears and to think more positively about my future. For the first time I am not anxious about my upcoming doctor's appointment.

In my Inner Healer exercise, there was a big wooden door that opened to a yellow light. The yellow light formed a winding path – it was my own healing path. I followed it – I was up in the air floating. It was so warm, peaceful and loving. Afterwards I felt I was still floating. I saw beauty everywhere: in traffic, city buildings, all around me.

My inner healer was my maternal grandmother. I've never met her but I know what she looks like from pictures. I've always felt a connection with her. When I got to the clearing and met her, it was very peaceful. I asked her if the chemo was going to work and she responded, "I do not know, but I want you to know that I love you." I had goose bumps all through me when I heard that. I have never felt love like that before. And then the love turned into a white light.

Further Practice and Study

Martin Rossman's books, Guided *Imagery for Self-Healing* and *Fighting Cancer from Within* are excellent resources. Guided imagery scripts and cds are also widely available. The Inner Healer exercise is available at www.healingjourney.ca. See books, videos and audio resources.

5. The Healing Light

What is it?

It is an exercise in evoking health, clarity, love, and comfort through imagining a healing light. For some it is a way of connecting to God or the divine.

How Is It Healing?

Cross cultures and over the millennia light has symbolized healing, clarity and divine spirit. In our culture, we "shed light" to gain understanding. We "see the light" in moments of transformation and we depict saints, as "shining forth with light" to show their pure qualities of holiness. In times of darkness, we "seek the light" at the end of the tunnel. We find sustenance in symbols of healing, hope and comfort: the white coat of medicine, a lotus flower, a heart, a butterfly or teddy bear. The symbol of healing light is perhaps the most accessible, powerful and deeply rooted of them all. We can use this to our advantage.

Tibetan Perspective on Healing Light

Tibetan Buddhism has a long history of seeing light as a powerful healing force and using imagery to evoke it. You can "awaken to this energy" and use it daily by simply noticing the light around you. Tulku Thondup suggests in *The Healing Power of Mind* to appreciate natural light as you go through your day. Notice the sunshine and the quality of light as it shifts and changes at different times of the day and night and in different seasons of the year. Use light as a metaphor for clarity, vitality and the free flow of energy and healing throughout your body. For example, imagine wellness in your body like a celebration of light and energy and clarity in your mind as a strong, clear and steady light.

Light as Healing Energy

Because light is such a universal symbol of wisdom, clarity and divine presence across many religions and cultures, it is ideally suited as a metaphor for personal transformation and healing. By conjuring light, you are drawing on this source of power. You imagine a beautiful healing light shining through every cell in your body, eliminating any toxins, stress, dysfunction or irregularity and replacing them with radiant health and vitality. Your body, mind and spirit open to the warmth, ease and peacefulness of total wellbeing.

Try It

- Close your eyes. Bring awareness to your breath, breathing in and out slowly, deeply and comfortably. As you breathe in, breathe in a sense of comfort. Imagine breathing in warmth, kindness and love. As you breathe out, let go of tension in your body and worries in your mind. Imagine releasing them more and more with each out breath. Relax into the rhythm of your breath . . . breathing in comfort, breathing out tension.

- Now picture a beautiful healing light above your head. This light embodies healing and all that is fine and good in the human spirit. Imagine this powerful and intelligent light streaming into you and around you. Your entire being is bathed in the beautiful light. Make this real and powerful for yourself in any way that feels right for you. See and feel the warm healing radiance filling every cell of your body and imagine every fibre of your being responding to the healing presence of this wonderful light.

- Imagine this energy eliminating all tension, worries and anxieties and replacing them with radiance, vitality and peace. Imagine feeling clear, calm, at peace. See it happen. Feel it happen. You might even hear it happen.

- Now feel a special concentration of this light gathering at your own heart centre – your heart opening and warming with compassion and love. Feel this radiating from your heart centre to others around you and then to the wider world – radiating warmth and care and peace.

- Sit quietly for a few moments before opening your eyes. Keep this clear, warm, harmonious feeling with you throughout your day.

I Can't Do It. I Can't See the Light.

Neither could I when I first started doing this exercise. Naturally I was concerned about this. How could I lead others in this exercise if I couldn't do it myself? It took me some time, but eventually I relaxed and I recognized that even though I could not see an image of light, I could feel light – a sensation of warmth moving through my body. With practice, I found I could direct this feeling of warmth to any part of my body and now, after years of doing this exercise, I actually see light. But the feeling of warmth is still the stronger sensation for me and it is the one I open into and relax most completely with. The key is to let go of expectations and notice what is happening as you relax your body and conjure light. Whatever you experience is fine – there is no right way or wrong way of doing the exercise. With time and practice, your experience will likely deepen and become meaningful for you.

Practice. Practice. Practice.

Practice this anywhere, anytime. You can do the exercise in a minute and use it while stuck in traffic, waiting for appointments or whenever you feel a flash of irritation or impatience. Or you can draw the exercise out, imagining every part of your body in great detail flooded with light. In moments of anxiety or worry, you can turn to the light for comfort and strength. Some people routinely use this exercise as a ritual before getting into a car or starting any journey. One person I know calms her fears about flying by sending the pilot light as she boards the plane and then envisioning the entire aircraft bathed in light. Other people find it is a powerful way of experiencing spiritual or religious connection.

I can think of light anytime and feel it wash through my body. I feel very close to God. I can feel His arms around my shoulders and His voice in my ear. I always feel His presence. When I'm tired, it's closer.

I imagine myself filled and surrounded with light as I step into the sea. Healing and goodness are all around me. Land, sea and sky all blend together. I feel at one with everything.

Further Practice and Study

Another way of working with light imagery is to recite the divine light invocation as meditation, mantrum or prayer. Like all the techniques introduced here, the more often you do it, the more powerful it becomes for you. For further instruction, consult Swami Radha's "The Divine Light Invocation".

Divine Light Invocation

I am created by divine light.

I am sustained by divine light.

I am protected by divine light.

I am surrounded by divine light.

I am ever growing into divine light.

Tulku Thondup's inspiring books *The Healing Power of Mind* and *Boundless Healing* also provide extensive instruction on using light and other imagery for healing.

Seven

Caregivers

For Partners, Family Members and Friends

This book is as much for you as for your loved one with cancer. In some ways, more so, because the significant load you are carrying is not always registered by the people around you as attention naturally centres on the cancer patient. Yet those words, "You have cancer" are often as disturbing for you as your loved one and the emotional roller coaster that follows, just as unsettling.

Your life has been changed. Not only is there the emotional upset, but there is also considerable upheaval in the day-to-day running of your family's life, which now has to accommodate a myriad of appointments, hospital visits and treatment schedules, plus the reassignment of who does what in household chores and management. Financial worries related to costs not covered by health plans, loss of work, and the myriad of expenses related to transport and care can also mount. At times you may go through the same ups and downs as the patient and at times they may be very different. Because so much of your experience is dependent on the patient's, you may feel unentitled to or confused by your own separate thoughts and feelings and repress them to better serve your loved one. Attention to your own needs and concerns then fall to the back burner. Resentment and fatigue can build. After a while, this is a recipe for burnout.

So how do you balance your need to do everything you possibly can for your loved one while still looking after yourself? There is no one magic formula, but I believe the strategies in this book on how to calm your mind and warm your heart provide the foundation for looking after yourself, managing the ups and downs of emotions and handling whatever comes your way.

How Can I Help Myself?

Read this book as if it is for you alone, not the cancer patient. Even though much of the material comes through the perspective of cancer patients, it still applies directly to you. Calming your mind means facing your own fears and learning strategies to manage your distressing thoughts more effectively. Warming your heart means letting go of anger, hurt and resentments and opening up to more peaceful and loving experiences, through greater acceptance, forgiveness and self help practices, such as meditation and journaling. Try all the techniques and find out which works most effectively for you. "Make it real" by integrating these practices into your life so that they make a difference. It can be as simple as learning to take a deep breath when you find yourself getting worked up and telling yourself, "I choose peace. Not this" or imagining a beautiful warm healing light washing over your body.

How Can I Help My Loved One With Cancer?

A key message in this book is the importance of warm-hearted connection with others for healing and general wellbeing. Yet at times of crisis, when we need it the most, we often retreat from such connection because we feel too tired, resentful or stressed. So taking care of yourself is an important factor in helping your loved one. If you don't look after yourself, you won't be much help to your partner, family member or friend with cancer.

• Calm Your Mind and Warm Your Heart

You will best help your family member or friend if you bring a calm mind and a warm heart to your interactions. Cancer brings a lot of changes into your life. It is natural to feel resentful at times. Be gentle with yourself when things weigh heavily upon you. Practice whatever techniques help you regain some comfort and peace. Cultivate loving kindness to yourself.

• Find Out What the Patient Considers Helpful

People vary tremendously in what they consider helpful. Some people are very independent and prefer to manage on their own as much as possible. Others welcome help. If you are a parent or the partner of a cancer patient, you will naturally be engaged in the care of your loved one and likely have a good idea about what is needed. If you are a friend or relative, the best way to help is not as clear. Figure out what you can do and make a specific offer. For example, you might offer to do some grocery shopping, pick up kids from school, walk the dog or mow the lawn. Many need help driving to and from appointments or supportive assistance in the actual appointment to record what is said and to help manage anxiety. Sometimes you can help by searching out specific information or resources for the patient. Often a friend or family member can be most helpful by simply listening in a supportive non judgmental way. If the patient declines your help, don't take it personally. Stay in touch, check in from time to time and signal you are still ready to help should the patient need it.

• Take Your Cues From the Patient

What is helpful one day may not be the next. Mood and energy levels can fluctuate greatly and influence the degree of support and care needed, so it is important to take your cues from the patient. One day they may want to talk about important issues, the next day to avoid them. One moment they may have energy to do things for themselves or others, the next moment, none. Fatigue is a key factor – cancer patients often say they wish there was a special term to describe their fatigue because the words in common usage don't capture their experience. Here is a common example: Kim and her husband were out together with friends. She was feeling great for the first two hours, but then fatigue struck "like a curtain coming down" and she needed to leave. She didn't want to spoil her husband's evening out, but she knew it would take all her energy simply to get home. "One moment you have energy, the next you have none." This abrupt change of plans can be hard on family members and friends who don't always understand how completely fatigue can take over and deplete the patient of resources.

- **Recognize Your Own Limits; Accept Help**

Accepting help from others is often difficult for patients and caregivers alike. As a caregiver, particularly for the partner or parent of a patient, there can be high expectations from all quarters, including yourself, that your new job is to meet every new demand the situation places upon you. People believe it's up to them to manage their own lives and they don't like imposing on others for assistance. Yet many of these same people would be the first to offer help to others in a similar situation. Use the guidance in this book to check in with yourself regularly. Monitor your stress levels in your body, mind and spirit. So often people wait until they are ready to collapse or explode before acknowledging they are stressed and need help with managing all the new circumstances and pressures cancer brings into the household. Recognize your own limits. It is better to say, "I can't do this right now" than to push yourself beyond your limits and create a climate of building stress and resentment. Learn to ask for help or to accept help that has been offered. Seek professional help if you feel consistently overwhelmed or depressed.

- **Try Not to Give Advice Unless You are Asked For It**

This is a tough one for most people. We have our own ideas about what is helpful and we press them upon the patient. Generally we do this because we care and we believe it is in the best interests of the patient. Often it also helps us to feel better because as long as something is being done, we can keep our worst thoughts at bay. Our advice may be sound and well worth heeding or it may be off base and unhelpful. Either way, we are not being supportive to the patient when we give unsolicited advice or direction.

Cancer patients are constantly told to "think positively." Diets or alternative therapies may be researched and pushed without the consent or interest of the patient. Mostly this is done out of care and love for the patient, but in so doing, caregivers risk pushing their own agendas and not listening to what the patient believes or considers important.

It can be very frustrating, even heart breaking, when we believe something will help an ill family member or friend, but he or she shows no interest and does not comply with our plan. As caregivers we can feel resentful that the patient doesn't do more to help themselves. It feels like they are just sitting back and accepting things rather than fighting or trying a new cure, or anything else that could improve the situation. Tension can really build around these issues.

The difficult truth is we can't change someone else or "fix" the problems of others. We can only change ourselves and model the behavior we would like to see in others. We can certainly communicate our hopes and wishes. Such expression is very important in loving and caring relationships. But we can't tell somebody else what to do.

The art of a supportive relationship is to communicate your hopes, wishes and beliefs in a way that clearly expresses their importance to you, while not enforcing them or directing others. For example, let's say your partner is feeling despondent and you want to cheer him up. Instead of saying, "just think positively," try reflecting back what you heard him say about these difficulties. "Yes it is hard when . . ." Listen without interrupting and continue to reflect back what you hear without giving advice. After you have really listened to his perspective, offer your own in a non directive, caring way. For example, you could say "When I'm feeling down, it helps me to think positively about things " or "I know it's difficult but, for me, it would be important to try . . ." Give examples from your own experience. In cases where you want your partner to try something new, instead of telling him he needs to do it for his own good, tell him what you know about this new course of action and ask him his thoughts about it. If he continues to show no interest, recognize there is not much you can do. Express your own hopes, and beliefs without resentment or blaming.

- ## Listen Supportively

Listening without interrupting or giving advice is a challenge for most of us. Yet it is one of the most supportive things we can do for someone else. To really listen, you need to give your full attention to what is being said instead of thinking ahead to what you are going to say next. Don't interrupt. Wait until the person has finished speaking before you start. Reflect back what you heard the person say. This is not as easy as it sounds. We tend to listen through our own filters, so reflecting back only what the person said, without our own additions or distortions, is hard to do. The reflecting back process shows you are listening and encourages the person to continue. You can further encourage a person by nodding your head and saying things like "Yes" "I see" or "Tell me more." If you are upset or confused by what is being said, it's okay and often helpful to acknowledge these feelings: "I'm doing my best, but I find this hard to hear" or "I'm trying to understand, but I'm feeling confused. Can you tell me more?" You can also check out your impressions: "From what you've said, I'm getting this impression . . . Is that right?" Try to withhold giving advice unless you are asked for it.

• Find Support for Yourself and Take Time Out

Who is there to listen to you in this way? Bottling up your emotions and keeping busy may help for a while, but in the long run, it is in your best interests of your own health and wellbeing to unburden your thoughts and feelings to someone who can really listen. Often this person is outside your family circle so you can talk freely without worrying about burdening them or the ties that may involve them in your situation. Sometimes there is no such person, so seeking out a support group, a counsellor or some form of spiritual or religious guidance can help.

It is also important to take a break from your situation to let off steam and escape your worries for a while. Exercising, walking in a park, going for a movie are all simple outings that you can work into your routine if you give it priority. The trouble is most people don't. Taking time for yourself is important for you and your family. Without time to replenish yourself, you are at risk of becoming tired, burned out and resentful and taking it out on the people around you.

- **Enjoy Time Together**

Cancer brings some couples closer together and wrenches others further apart. Hopefully the guidance in this book related to calming your mind and warming your heart will help you make choices that move you toward enjoying time together without the constant wrench of cancer. Make a point of bringing some fun into your lives by going on outings, renting funny movies and enjoying time with family and friends. Sometimes the crisis of cancer renews a couple's love through the reformulating of what is important in life. Maggie's case was unusual. First she was diagnosed with advanced cancer and then her husband had a heart attack amid her cancer crisis.

It took cancer and a heart attack to make us realize what is and what is not important. Family is important. Material things are not important. Life isn't just career and making money. My husband and I are talking again as we did when we first met. We're talking and getting to know each other again. There's a certain excitement as if life is starting to open again. We are going out for a date tonight and I feel like a kid again. I feel like I'm dating again. Our kids notice we're different, more affectionate with one another. It's rubbing off on them. They're getting along better too.

- **Recognize "Back to Normal" is Not That Simple**

Wanting things to be "back to normal" is a yearning commonly expressed by cancer patient and caregiver alike. They want their old lives back and count down the weeks and days until the end of treatment. Yet getting "back to normal" may not be as simple as it sounds. Caregivers often expect that once treatment is over, life will instantly go back to the way it was before cancer. But for cancer patients the end of treatment can be an especially vulnerable time – during treatment there is the comfortable sense that everything is being done to fight the cancer, but when treatment ends, the abrupt cut off from regular medical attention can leave them feeling anxious rather than relieved. Often too the patient is emotionally and physically exhausted and so while family and friends celebrate the end of treatment, the patient may feel exhausted and numb. Once treatment stops, patients have more time to reflect upon their illness and what it has meant for them and their families. They may feel changed by the experience and find "getting back to normal" more complicated than they expected. It is helpful if both caregivers and patients give themselves time and flexibility to recover and make sense of the experience, rather than expect an instant return to the old way of life.

End of Life Issues

The next chapter describes the particular challenges of living with advanced cancer and end of life issues, mostly from the patient's perspective. For caregivers too, this is an especially difficult and challenging time.

Anticipatory Grief

When a partner, family member or friend is nearing the end of life, the thought of losing them is naturally very much on your mind. You may begin to grieve their loss and think ahead to how life will be without them. Sometimes people feel guilty about this. They criticize themselves for imagining their loved ones gone when they are still living and feel ashamed of the thoughts as if they represent some failure in their capacity to love and support their loved one.

Grief can be overwhelming and it is natural to anticipate and begin to prepare for your loss. Some people, both patients and caregivers, are able to talk openly about the subject and this can bring tremendous comfort to people in both situations. The benefits of talking openly together are covered elsewhere in this book. The point emphasized here is that there no reason to feel guilty or ashamed if you are privately jumping ahead and anticipating your loss and your life without your loved one. There is some benefit in beginning to approach and understand the challenges, emotionally and circumstantially, that await you.

A patient living with advanced cancer once asked me to see her husband privately because she was concerned about how he was going to cope without her. Her greatest fear about dying was that her husband would collapse into depression and live a miserable existence. Whenever she brought up the topic, he shut down completely and only reiterated, he couldn't live without her. When he came to see me, he told me he spent a lot of time thinking about what it would be like when his wife died. He felt very guilty about these thoughts, which he considered dis-loyal. He loved his wife and he worried these thoughts meant he wanted to hasten her death. He knew he was going to be okay, but he couldn't tell his wife that because it felt so disloyal. He was staggered to learn that what she needed most from him was the one thing he avidly kept from her: this acknowledgement that he would be okay. They sorted this out. They were each able to express their love for the other and his reassurance that he was going to be okay allowed her to die peacefully.

Burnout

The long drawn out nature of living with chronic illness, par-ticularly advanced illness can tax both patients and partners and desensitize others. Remarks like the following usually draw a knowing laugh in support groups:

The first month everyone calls. Two or three years later, it's like "Are you staying or are you going?"

I remember a very touching interchange between two women, both of whom were considered to be close to the end of their lives by medical evaluation, but continued to live nonetheless. One asked the other, "Does your husband ever . . ." She paused, clearing having trouble saying the words. The other woman supplied them for her "Wish it was over?" They both acknowledged that this was often the case. "Part of him wishes it was over. It's harder for him to see me in pain than for me to experience the pain." The other believed her husband was taxed by repeated crises, hospital visits and anticipatory grief. He was worn out physically and emotionally and now longed for the cer-tainty of an endpoint.

It is hard to go on and on living in this precarious uncertain way. Living with uncertainty is difficult at the best of times and even more complex and taxing at the end of life when you expect the end may be a matter of days, but weeks and even months go by. It is natural to be both heartened and disheart-ened by the extra time when you are feeling worn out by the cir-cumstances and saddened by your grief. But even in these most difficult times it is possible to have special, even transcendent moments when suffering opens into warm-hearted connection, when people openly and authentically express their love and care for one another. The next chapter describes several such moments amid all the challenges of living with advanced illness.

Eight
Living with Advanced Cancer

I'm a hell of a survivor. Stats aren't meant for me.

Live because you want to live, not because you fear death

When and how I die is beyond my control. But I have resources to manage my fears. I can control how I respond to the things that weigh heavily on me. I don't want a fear of death to control the way I live my life. I want to live from a place of strength, not a place of fear. I have a strong will to live.

In July 1945, an American naval ship, the USS Indianapolis, was torpedoed by a Japanese submarine, a few weeks before the end of World War 11. The ship capsized and sank in twelve minutes with more than 1000 men on board. Survivors waited in the water for days, not knowing if rescue would appear. Not only did they have to deal with dehydration and exposure, but they were also terrorized by regular shark attacks, targeting some of the men.

Jake, a middle aged man living with advanced prostate cancer, could relate to this story. It had elements of his own experience – hit out of nowhere by cancer, stranded and uncertain about rescue, frightened and demoralized by his situation and all the while having to contend with his worst fear – the possibility of a shark lurking under the surface, ready to strike.

It is challenging enough to deal with the news "You have cancer." It is devastating to learn there is no curative medical treatment for your disease. It takes a while to assimilate such news, your mind in a whirl, your spirit rising and falling with the ebb and flow of hope and despair. Often there are still many treatment options that may successfully diminish symptoms and keep your disease stable for several years or longer. Even when all options are exhausted, there is still hope of living fully and meaningfully in whatever time you have left. Some cancer patients respond to the news as a rallying call – they are determined to beat the odds and show the doctors they are wrong. They find sustenance and spirit in their determination to live. Others find strength in accepting the news and living their lives in ways that affirm what is most important to them. This chapter charts the ups and downs of living with advanced cancer through challenging issues, such as accepting versus fighting the cancer, anxiety about planning, finding meaning and humor, dealing with pain and debilitation, and facing death.

Feeling Frightened and Abandoned

When Jake recounted the USS Indianapolis story, he was no longer feeling frightened and abandoned. The key for him was to live his life without feeling intimidated by "the shark." This meant facing his fears and drawing on his own resources for comfort and peace:

If you constantly live in fear of the shark coming back, you're sunk. You need strong management of your mind and your emotions to combat that paralyzing fear. Sometimes, fear grips me in the middle of the night. I've worked hard at finding a peaceful place within to help me through those times. I've also prayed all my life. But I wouldn't pray to save me from the sharks. I pray for strength and peace because I think help comes through me, through this inner peaceful place.

Recognizing that death is part of life and something we all eventually face helped Jake face his fears and affirm his belief that life is for living, not for waiting to die.

These days I feel more at ease. It's not just about me. That was a revelation. We all have a death sentence. Maybe the hill is a little steeper for me. But it is nothing different than what everyone faces or will face. You acknowledge these fears and live with them. Live because you want to live, not because you fear death. Don't live waiting to die. It was an important thing for me to learn – to live, but not to live out of desperation.

In the early days of assimilating difficult news, peace of mind can seem a long way off. In addition to fear, it is not uncommon to feel abandoned and alone. Some patients feel their doctors "write them off." Others feel apart and discarded by a world that continues to hum along in its busy ways, oblivious to their plight. Even members of support groups sometimes believe they will no longer be welcome at their support meetings because their news sets them apart and will discourage others. Over time, these feelings usually settle – but not without first causing significant distress.

I'm angry with doctors who just throw their hands in the air and say "That's it. There's nothing more we can do." Sure they don't have a treatment, but they don't make any suggestions about what you can do. They just leave you on your own. If you don't ask the right questions, you have no idea of what help you can get. It would be so useful if they had a list and would say, "This is what other people have tried in your situation, maybe one of these resources will help you." If it isn't within their expertise or beliefs, then they won't talk about it. It doesn't matter that a person's life is on the line. They simply send you on your journey toward death without a map.

Learning you have an incurable disease is devastating, but the devastation is made even worse when the people you believe in seem to abandon you to your fate.

Finding Hope

"It's hard to find hope when the doctors give you none.

For many hope means cure. Having hope means believing you can get well again. When you are told there is no longer curative treatment, the stakes get higher. It is harder to hold on to this hope when the doctors give you none. What does hope mean then?

Many respond to a diagnosis of incurable cancer with a strong fighting stance. They are fighting for their lives and they are determined to win. This determination often serves them well – they find hope and spirit in their vision of wellness. I admire this spirit and I believe it can make a difference in the course of cancer. I know the human mind is a powerful tool in the healing process. But I also know there are no guarantees. If hope only means cure for you, then you have a tight grip on one outcome and you restrict your ability to find hope in other places and perspectives.

I believe there is always hope and hope goes well beyond the possibility of getting well again. No matter what you face in your cancer prognosis, no matter how you are feeling at the moment, there is always the possibility of lightening your load through opening your heart and spirit to a wider perspective than the fearful one holding you in its grip. Hope counterbalances fear. For Jake, hope was connecting with his own resources for "strength and peace" to live his life without being controlled by fear.

This book is essentially about finding hope through the practices of calming your mind and warming your heart. When you calm your mind and warm your heart, you exert your own capacity to live fully, no matter what you face. That is hope in a nutshell. But can such practices change the course of advanced cancer? Can hope still include getting well when you are facing this tough prognosis?

Can the Mind Heal the Body?

There is always hope that these practices will help you fare better than predicted. I have personally seen several examples of "spontaneous remission" in which advanced cancers have disappeared and many more cases where people lived long past the limited time spans predicted for them. But there is no magic formula and certainly no guarantees of making any difference on the course of illness.

Our research at the Healing Journey Program at Princess Margaret Hospital in Toronto investigated the question of whether engaging in self-help practices can extend the survival time of cancer patients. Our results were not conclusive – an early study found a strong relationship between the degree of engagement in self-help activity (such as meditation, journaling, imagery and spiritual work) and survival time, but further research did not present such a clear cut picture. For a complete report and analysis, refer to Alastair Cunningham's book, *Can the Mind Heal Cancer?* Some relevant research papers are also available online at www.healingjourney.ca.

As a past researcher and clinician at the Healing Journey Program, I believe that engaging in self help practices, such as the ones advocated in this book, gives you the best chance of extending your life and achieving greater peace of mind. I believe too there is always the possibility of physical cure. But there is also the very real possibility that no matter what you do the disease will progress as predicted. Your self-help practices will stand you in good stead just the same – they can help you find hope, peace, and comfort no matter what you are facing.

Accepting Versus Fighting the Illness

I'm fighting for my life and I'll fight to the last.

Many struggle with the dilemma of whether to fight or accept their illness. Those with a strong fighting stance hold firmly to their belief that they can beat their cancer. Anything that challenges this is viewed as threatening. This usually means they have tight control over their emotions as they need to repress any doubts or fears to maintain their spirit. Typically they have high energy, a strong commitment to their beliefs and inspire hope in others. Challenging news or new symptoms can set them back for a while, but soon they regain their spirit to fight on. Such spirit is remarkable and inspiring. However sometimes it comes with a cost – the need to appear upbeat and well restricts the range of opportunities for help and care from others, even when changing circumstances require it. Disclosure is usually tightly controlled so the people who care about these patients, either don't know the full extent of what they are facing or don't feel they are allowed to talk about it.

Martha was a case in point. If I had to choose one word to describe Martha it would be "indomitable." She had risen through the ranks of corporate structure to a prominent position. She had clear organizational and management skills and moved through life with an efficient To Do list. She had the same confident approach to illness and her personal life. She was going to beat the disease and she allowed no other option. She protected her children and husband from the difficult aspects of illness, by always maintaining she was well, even when she wasn't, by discounting any need for help and by the sheer force of her considerable willpower. She knew she had tight control of things, but that's how she liked it.

When her disease progressed, she continued to exert control. She was taken aback when a close friend told her she felt "shut out" and asked her to be more open and honest about what was happening to her. She acknowledged similar messages from her husband and fellow group members. But then her customary vigor and confidence returned. She asked herself, "could they all be wrong?" Her response was a defiant, "Yes."

Martha's fierce determination formed the solid core of her fighting spirit and made her remarkably resilient. Her own near death experience changed her perspective from tight control toward greater openness and acceptance. It will be fully described later. A fitting testament to her remarkable spirit, Martha is the only person I know who actually cancelled her own funeral!

Greater Acceptance Does Not Mean "Giving up"

Just because I accept that death may come to me sooner than later, doesn't mean I'm giving up. Acceptance gives me a firm base to be open and active.

This is an important point that some "fighters" miss: accepting the possibility that death may come sooner than later, does not mean giving up hope. You can hold both – the hope of getting better and the possibility you may die. Life, after all, is a terminal condition. As Jake says, sooner or later, we all face a death sentence. Looking it in the eye helps to loosen the tight grip fear can have over you. Paradoxically facing death is what affirms life. It frees you to live life with meaning. It gives you a firm base to be open and active and to live your life in a way that calms your mind, warms your heart and affirms what is most meaningful to you. You can be open and accepting and still embrace a "fighting spirit."

It's about accepting what is. That's really where the struggle is. Once you do that there's no guilt. There's no blame. It just is. When you accept that, you clear the table of all those feelings, all that fear.

Louise, a young mother living with metastatic breast cancer, was the principal income earner in her family. Her main struggle revolved around this question of whether accepting she might die meant giving in to her illness. She needed to be doing everything she possibly could to beat the disease and be around for her daughter and husband. She did not want to "give in" in any sense. After being in our Healing Journey research program for a year, she noticed changes in herself – she was able to calm her mind through the practice of meditation and warm her heart by being more open and receptive to the world around her and by listening to her inner voice. She felt more at peace and began to experience a spiritual connection with "something bigger" than herself. She found that holding on tightly to the need for physical cure became an obstacle because it was steeped in fear and fear "occupies a big space." She began to understand that healing could extend beyond physical cure to encompass changes in body, mind and spirit and "the ultimate healing is having peace of mind." Accepting that did not change her determination to get better, rather it helped it by giving her new perspective on how to manage her fears.

I came to this program for healing and that meant for me: physical healing – curing my disease. But now I see that healing encompasses body, mind and spirit and there is more to healing than physical cure. For example, I've come to rely on meditation. When I feel my mind starting to churn, I can break the cycle – even ten minutes of meditation helps me get my focus back and feel grounded again. For the past year, I've been more in touch with my inner voice and I've made better decisions and been more open and receptive. It has helped me evolve spiritually. I still feel like I'm taking baby steps and I haven't found the words that I'm comfortable with yet – but I do feel very powerfully a strong connection to something bigger than myself.

I think if physically healing continued to be my only reason for doing this, it would somehow be empty of its real meaning. I've had to accept the uncertainty of whether or not I'm going to achieve physical healing. I found that question was creating a big obstacle for me because it is such a huge question: "Can I get well again?" At first it was my motivation, I came here for physical healing, but then it became an obstacle. Because when that question is in my mind, what takes over is fear. Fear occupies a big space. It doesn't allow peace to enter.

So now I look at healing in this broader sense and I believe the ultimate healing is having peace of mind. What I wrestle with sometimes is whether this means I'm giving in to the illness? How can you have peace of mind when you're facing this? But I don't see it as giving into the illness at all. I see it as accepting the uncertainty. I haven't accepted that because I have metastatic breast cancer that I'm going to die, but I have accepted that I don't have total control and no matter what I do, it is uncertain what the outcome will be.

Living Life With Meaning

When life is threatened, it becomes more precious. Cancer brings an opportunity to consider important questions – what is the meaning of my life? How might I live my life fully? What values are most important to me? What changes do I need to make to live in accordance with these values?

Sometimes the opposite occurs – when life is threatened, it loses meaning. Such was the case for a middle aged man who came to our support group for people living with metastatic cancer at Wellspring. It was his first visit and he looked glum.

He told us his cancer had spread and that there was no longer curative treatment available to him. He loved music, but could no longer listen to it. He retreated from time with family and friends. He kept asking himself, "What's the point? What's the point?" Group members offered him support and encouragement, but he continued to look glum. They told their own stories about how they found meaning – living the moment, travelling, spending time with loved ones, creative expression, finding peace and comfort through meditation and spiritual connection. The stories would have gone on, but he interrupted them and insisted that they didn't understand – he had been told there was no cure for his disease. They nodded their heads. Many of them had been told the same thing. He looked puzzled. He related more details of his difficult situation and again they nodded their heads. It finally dawned on him that most everyone in the room was facing similar circumstances and yet they were enjoying life, spending time with family and friends and laughing easily. He started to smile. At the end of the group, he said "I really like your attitude! I can see it makes all the difference." He left with a spring in his step.

How Do You Get Comfortable With This?

You may not be going around saying "What's the point? What's the point?" but you may be haunted nonetheless by the question "How do I get comfortable with this?" As Louise put it "How can you have peace of mind when you're facing serious cancer?"

Finding a reason to get up in the morning with a spring in your step can be a challenge. Knowing what feeds and dampens your spirit is a good place to start in your quest to live your day in a way that reflects what is most important and meaningful to you. In chapter five we listed many responses to the question, "What opens and enriches your spirit?" You may want to review the list to remind yourself of what resonates most immediately with you. Often people look for a Big answer to the question of "What is the meaning of my life?" But I suspect the answer can be simple as choosing to live your life with a calm mind and warm heart. I hope this book has provided some guidance along those lines. Even so, it is one thing to have a "guide" in hand, it is another to have a "spring in your step."

Live the Moment

I don't focus on the future. It's enough to have one good day. One good day may lead to another good day. Your whole life in this one day. The past doesn't exist – the future who knows? If I'm able to live one good day, I can be content.

Many find comfort by taking one day at a time. So much suffering comes from ruminating on past problems or future worries, that you miss opportunities to enjoy the present moment. Learning to take a day at a time focuses your energy to engage with life as it is unfolding now. When you bring full awareness to the present moment, you exercise your potential to live joyfully. The present moment is all we ever have. The future is always one moment ahead, the past always one moment behind. We live and breathe the present moment. This very simple truth contains a recipe for happiness. Eckhart Tolle spells it out clearly and simply in his bestselling book, *The Power of Now*. When we bring mindful awareness to "Now," without judging it as "good" or "bad" or bringing our own expectations of how things "should" be and accept the moment as it is, then we let go of all the suffering associated with our own distortions. We become more aware of our peaceful core, or "presence" – that part of us that never changes.

Spiritual Connection

Such mindful awareness often brings a spiritual connection that helps people handle their illness with greater peace and equanimity:

For me spirituality means to bring the sacred into everyday life; to live in a state of awareness as much as possible; to treat every relationship as a new opportunity to really listen, make contact, give love, regardless of the emotions I may be feeling; to go inside myself and find a still peaceful place each day. I now spend much more of my time in spiritual practices and that has really helped me to learn to face and accept what is happening to me. It has helped me to feel more hopeful that I can handle whatever happens with equanimity and to be less fearful that all the worst things I can imagine will happen. It has helped me to shift my focus away from myself and cancer to others and the outside world. I see myself as part of something bigger now, and less of an isolated being with a serious problem.

My spiritual path evolved around nature and the continuity of nature. I like the wave image in the book Tuesdays with Morrie. *I'm not just a single wave about to crash into the shore and become nothing. I'm also part of the ocean. I'm both the wave and the ocean. It does not bother me if there's no life after death. I won't care. What is important to me is awareness in this moment. It's time that gives us the fixation with the afterlife. If we just live each moment, it would be healthier. I think it's important to live life with reverence.*

People with strong religious beliefs find significant comfort in their religious convictions, practices and community. It serves them well when they need it the most. Their beliefs give meaning to their lives and they feel loved, protected and cared for, no matter what happens. Some feel abandoned by God and need to work through these feelings before they can reconnect with their beliefs. Others want to turn to religion for comfort, but their own critical minds stop them – they believe that turning to religion only at a time of need undermines the sincerity and credibility of the intention.

Many have negative associations with religion or no interest in religious doctrine. Louise, the young mother mentioned earlier, was brought up to scoff at religion: her father used to joke that Jesus Christ would need to appear on the hood of his car before he'd believe. So it surprised Louise that her self help practices brought her more and more in touch with a core of peacefulness and the spiritual sense that she was connected with "something bigger" than herself.

Spiritual connection is based on personal experience, not religious doctrine. Louise started reading books recommended by other group members and through this reading and her own meditation practice, she felt drawn to incorporating prayer, and healing light imagery into her daily routines. "It was very calming and really gave me a lot of strength." The whole process "felt right." As she opened more and more to feelings of loving acceptance, she began to trust that "no matter what happens my life is going to work out as it should." With this growing trust, came less anxiety about her situation.

Peaceful Place Within

Spiritual connection is an expanding awareness of your own peaceful core. The practices in this book reinforce that process. As you learn to to calm your mind and warm your heart, you become more able to access that peacefulness and to live with meaning and joy, no matter what you face. Some of the participants in our program radiated an inner peace and spirit that touched and influenced everyone they met. As researchers, we tried to define it, but it was hard to pin down. They seemed to "glow"; they were at ease with themselves and their situation and they brought clarity, wisdom, humor and spirit to our weekly meetings. They had many different ways of expressing what was meaningful to them and how they integrated and practiced their spiritual awareness. Some felt a personal connection to God or the divine, others did not. They all had in common a powerful feeling that no matter what happened, things would be okay. There were many others in our weekly sessions who did not share this confidence or "knowing," but were nonetheless comforted by the example of those that did. They were an inspiration to us all.

Struggle to Maintain Peaceful Perspective at Challenging Times

Whatever peace you have made with what is happening to you may be difficult to maintain at challenging times: when you feel overcome by sadness, when disease worsens, at times of pain. Just when you feel you've got a handle on things, the rug can be pulled out from under you and you find yourself struggling again. This is the nature of living with illness and the effort to get comfortable with it – you repeatedly face challenges in body, mind and spirit and you need to learn and re-learn your way through them. As one woman said, "We're always living on the edge." Here is another woman's description of the "emotional roller coaster":

Chemo is no longer working for me and fluid is building in my lungs. Just when I crawl back up, I get knocked down again. It's all so scary. It's all coming back again. I'm struggling to breathe and I'm just laying low. We all go through these stages of ups and downs – it is such an emotional roller coaster. Right now, it's a trough. I'm in shock and trying to absorb everything. I work hard but I still go down again. I hope not to stay down. I've climbed the hill before. I'll climb back up again.

Sometimes it feels like too much. The relentless nature of the disease is overwhelming and all a person wants is to have an end to all the suffering:

Is it really worth it? All this surgery, chemo, pain and hassle? Is life worth all this suffering?

Some do find an ability to remain calm despite worsening conditions. You can't expect this of yourself all the time, but it is helpful to know that it is possible. One woman remained calm while she struggled to breathe in the emergency room waiting for a procedure to drain fluid from her lungs. We asked her how she did it:

It's a horrible feeling not being able to breathe. I stay calm. I tell myself that if I panic, it will just make things worse. I've learned to face whatever I have to face. It's in my nature to be meditative and optimistic.

For some getting through difficult times is a matter of reconnecting with their fighting spirit or will to live. For others, it is connecting with their peaceful place and drawing on their inner resources:

I'm going to fight to the end. I'm not finished yet. I don't think about these new symptoms too much. They don't bother me anymore. I feel very calm. I want to live forever. I feel close to the people around me and I don't want to leave them. There's more to explore. I'm doing everything I can so there's no point worrying.

Even though doctors give me little time, I've survived before when others expected me to die. I don't rule out this happening again. I had a great summer. I'd like to make another Christmas.

When things get tough, I'm guided by three teachings: 1) listen to what my body tells me; 2) practice forgiveness and 3) be joyful.

Even when there is no longer hope of further treatment, there is the hope of maintaining peace of mind:

I can't have any more treatment because it will kill me. I still don't feel down. I have a lot of hope and prayers. I almost died a number of times and I'm still here. I've got to be here for a purpose. I feel in tune with my body. I check in with myself, asking "Is it time to die yet?" I feel it is not my time.

When I check in with myself, I feel a surge of energy wash over me. I feel recharged and positive. I have tremendous support from friends and community. When I nearly died, I felt floating in light, enveloped in light. I'm not afraid.

Pain and Nausea

Nothing undermines a spring in one's step as effectively as pain and nausea. It is hard to feel hopeful and peaceful in the midst of pain and discomfort. Not only is it hard to endure, but it brings the uncomfortable reminder that you are ill and the fear that things may be getting worse. Pain presents on a broad spectrum, and is experienced differently by different people. You are the best judge of the severity of your pain and discomfort.

Some people go to great lengths to deny their pain. Acknowledging it means "giving in to the illness" and they believe that as long as they are managing on their own, without the help of pills, then the cancer can't be that bad. Some fear that taking medication is a "downward spiral": taking pain control means they have started on an entirely new path, one that is likely to get worse, not better. Still others worry about getting addicted to pain medication or "masking symptoms" so they won't know the true picture of what is happening to them.

These worries are very common and get in the way of seeking help that can make a meaningful difference to the comfort and wellbeing of your mind, body and spirit. In a support group you learn how common these worries are and how others managed their way through them. You learn that opting for pain control does not mean you are on a downward spiral, nor does it mean you will become addicted to pain killers. You learn the pros and cons of taking medication and some of the side effects you may experience. And even though there is no one solution that works for everyone, most people who decide to seek out help for their pain are glad they did. They usually wonder why they waited so long.

Before, I was fighting against my pain, calling it "discomfort" and not taking pills. Now I realize I was robbing myself of the chance to feel better. I've learned to take pain medication proactively.

Some find that their self help practices stand them in good stead when they are in pain. They can find some relief through relaxation, meditation and imagery exercises. Others find nothing helps. Naturally they feel discouraged that when they need them the most, these practices are not useful to them – either they are in too much pain to do them or they do them and experience little relief. If you can, be gentle with yourself at these times. Accept that this is going to be one of those days where nothing seems to help. Reciting the mantra, "This too shall pass. This too shall pass" may offer you some sort of hope and support.

Meditation was the only thing that helped when I was in pain.

I try to ignore pain by keeping busy.

I don't know how you deal with pain. It feels like I'm sawed in half. Pain is frightening. It's out of control. It brings me down. It makes me wonder, 'What is it for? Why am I going through this?' It brings me closer to death.

Thoughts About Death:

You kind of come to terms with the fact you're going to die one day. You always hope for a good outcome, but you know things can change. There's still hope for more time, a last minute reprieve, a peaceful death.

I wonder if there's a point when I give up the struggle not to die and shift to dying gracefully?

Periods of sadness, pain, new symptoms can all bring thoughts of death to the surface. When a member dies in a support group, there is not only the loss to grieve, but also the sharp reminder of shared vulnerability and the unavoidable highlighting of one's own uncertain future.

When Sandy died, I had to separate my sadness at her passing from what I might be feeling about my own future. Am I feeling sad about this because it brings my own death into sharper focus? That was an important question to ask myself.

What is Most On Your Mind?

When thoughts of death come to the fore, it is natural to repress them. The thinking is, "Why go there now? It will only make me sad. I'll deal with this when I need to." That strategy makes a lot of sense and combined with whatever self help practices work for you – meditation, relaxation, imagery or journaling, it is possible to regain feelings of comfort and peace.

But there is also good reason to face your fears when you feel ready to do so. Asking yourself, "What is my worst fear about dying?" helps you identify what is most on your mind. Once you do that, you can address what you can do to put your mind at ease. Is there anything you need to know or put in place for your own or your family's peace of mind?

Seeking out a qualified palliative care professional to guide you through these thoughts and concerns is very helpful. People, who are feeling well, are often reluctant to make use of these opportunities because end of life issues seem a long way off and don't apply to them. There may be a superstitious thought that seeking out such assistance will hasten the need for it. But palliative care extends well beyond immediate care for the dying. Trained counsellors are excellent resources for helping you manage your situation more effectively and providing support and guidance for you and your family.

For example, when people face their greatest fear, they often find it is not so much about death, as about dying. The unknown nature of what lies ahead causes considerable anxiety. Concern about suffering and pain is frightening. Talking with your doctor or palliative care professional can really help:

I talked to my oncologist about my fears around dying. I wanted to know how I'm going to die and how we will manage pain. I like to know what's coming down the road. I was surprised by his comforting words. His care and reassurance made a huge difference.

One woman's greatest fear was dying alone. She had a nightmarish scenario in which she envisioned herself home alone and no one finding her for days. Expressing her fear helped her to make plans and seek out resources that gave her peace of mind.

Leaving Loved Ones

This is the hardest one to contemplate and the source of great sadness. Sometimes cancer patients express gratitude that they have had the time to reflect on their lives and find meaning and joy in living. They have opportunities to let loved ones know what they mean to them and to forgive and let go of unresolved hurts. People who die suddenly don't have this chance.

Cancer has given me time to make sense of things, find meaning in my life and to make changes so I feel more peaceful. I feel grateful for the time. People who die suddenly don't have that chance.

The sadness of leaving loved ones and missing out on important occasions can be overwhelming at times. Birthdays, holidays, and family outings all come tinged with the ache of: "Will I be here next year. Is this the last one?" Partners worry about how their "other half" will fare without them – adult children wonder who will care for their aging parents and support and love their siblings. Parents mourn the thought of missing the graduations, weddings and important events of their children's lives and the births of grandchildren. Parents of young children wonder who could ever love their children as much as they do and grieve for their futures without this guiding and encompassing love. In support groups, this grief, this ache, is palpably felt in the room. We all feel this sadness together.

There is no way of "fixing" or reframing this sadness. It is there, part of the bittersweet texture of feeling and expressing love. It is woven into the texture of close relationships and surfaces in many forms. One young mother described the sudden physical pain she experienced when her son innocently asked about their summer plans. She didn't know whether she'd be well enough to make any plans for the present summer and she was uncertain about whether she'd live to see another one. "The question was like a stone on my chest. I told him "We'll see. Let's take one day at a time."

Some people find comfort in their spiritual or religious beliefs. Expanding awareness of their own peaceful core can hold pain of this kind and lighten its load. Some have glimpses, others firmer footing, in a belief that knows, no matter what happens, things will be okay.

Special Projects

Working on special projects – journals, photo albums, videos, quilts – for their children help some parents with their feelings of loss. At first it is hard to get started since the project is so directly associated with their grief about possibly leaving their children, but once they start, they usually find the process eases their burden rather than adds to it. These projects take many different forms. One mother recorded day-to-day events in her relationship with her daughter, what they did together, and any special events or achievements. Her young daughter knew about this book and took great interest in it, knowing she was to receive it on her sixteenth birthday. One day she burst through the door after attending a Brownies meeting, proudly carrying a new badge. "Put it in the book, Mommy. I want you put it into your book!" The mother hopes she will be around to present "the book" to her daughter on her sixteenth birthday, but if she's not, she's glad there will be a record of their life together, for her daughter to enjoy and cherish.

Another mother I know anticipated important events in her children's lives – starting a new school, a first date, going off to university, their weddings and wrote notes for each of these events. "It was very hard to get started. But one day, I just did it. Now I enjoy the writing – it makes me feel good. I find it helpful."

One parent did not like the idea of writing, but arranged for someone to videotape herself reading stories to her young son and chatting with him about the story. It helped her to know that no matter what happened to her, there would be a record of this moment of story reading and shared fun and intimacy. Others make photo albums for their children writing notes and jotting thoughts as a way of connecting with their children and leaving a meaningful legacy. Creative projects – making a quilt, a stained glass window, a piece of art, are all ways that can comfort a parent by creating something personal and meaningful for their children.

Planning

Other issues that bring up considerable anxiety relate to planning – making wills, organizing funeral service and discussing wishes for burial or cremation. Some put it off, not ready to encounter the considerable hurdles of acknowledging life may be shortened or the sadness of leaving loved ones. Those that do it encourage others to follow suit because they experience tremendous relief it is done and they can now enjoy their lives without carrying this burden of unfinished business. They argue that taking care of such practical matters is not necessarily an end of life issue, but good planning practice for any responsible adult.

One woman marveled at the transition in herself over the years since her original diagnosis. When she first learned she had cancer, she could not talk about her fears to anyone and never acknowledged to herself or anyone else that she could die. But now she feels more at peace with life and death, she feels lighter in herself and more open and joyful with the world around her. Far from not being able to talk about her death, she told her husband the outfit she wanted to be buried in and joked with him, "If I'm too fat, just slit the back!"

Finding Humor, Even in Death

Many people find such humor macabre and in bad taste. But from my experience, I can attest to the therapeutic power of black humor and laughing at the unlaughable. In difficult moments, it opens us up and reconnects us with spirit. It brings light to the darkest moments and joins people together when they might otherwise feel sad, isolated, and apart. My mother tells the story of going to visit a friend dying of ovarian cancer. Her belly was swollen with ascites, a build-up of excessive fluid in the abdomen. My mother was shocked and saddened to see her friend this way and didn't know what to say. Her friend looked at her belly and said, "I just wish I knew who the father was!" The two friends laughed uproariously together like the old friends they were and conversation flowed from there.

When Graham Chapman died, his friend and fellow comedian from Monty Python, John Cleese, gave the eulogy at his memorial sevice. His speech started this way:

> Graham Chapman, co-author of the Parrot Sketch, is no more. He has ceased to be, bereft of life, he rests in peace, he has kicked the bucket, hopped the twig, bit the dust, snuffed it, breathed his last, and gone to meet the Great Head of Light Entertainment in the sky.

The service ended, with another Monty Python comedian, Eric Idle, leading the mourners in joyous singing of "Always look on the bright side of life." A viewer, not knowing the context, might well mistake the actual funeral for a comedy skit, but no one can doubt the warm, loving and celebratory nature of this spirited service.

Several of the people I have worked with have also showed remarkable spirit and openness toward the end of their lives. I got a phone call one afternoon informing me that a patient I had known for many years had been admitted to the hospital and was expected to die shortly. I went up to see her. She was only a short elevator ride away. I knew which floor she was on, but I didn't know her room number. As the elevator doors opened, I heard raucous laughter rolling out of one of the rooms and I knew that would be Jessie's room.

There was Jessie lying in bed, looking pale, but still laughing heartily with her husband. Under her bed, hidden from view was her beloved dog, a beautiful Labrador retriever. Jessie explained how hard it was for her to say goodbye to Ruff, this dog who meant so much to her. So her husband had pretended to be blind and had walked through the hospital stumbling along as if he couldn't see, letting Ruff guide him. The ruse had worked and Ruff was now safely stowed under the bed – his presence clearly given away by the rhythmic thump of his tail in tune to their laughter.

Jessie had predicted a year earlier that she would be cracking jokes on her deathbed and she was. I could only marvel at her spirit and join in with the laughter, joy and sadness in that room. Everyone in the group loved Jessie, her open, affectionate, joyful personality left an impression on us all and we aspired to be like her to the extent we could. Her big open heart never closed, even at the most difficult times. We had laughed and cried with her on many occasions and she was always ready to comfort and support others, no matter what she was going through. I remember the time her hair was falling out in big clumps because of yet another chemo regimen. She was saddened by this loss and all the other losses she had endured. Then she had an idea. She went out to her garden and threw chunks of her hair into the air, calling out to the birds, inviting them to use it for their nests. She laughed to think what she must have looked like to all the neighbors. We laughed right along with her. The ritual had made her feel better and she in turn had made all of us feel better. Her laughter and spirit were contagious. She lived life to the fullest with a warm, open and joyful heart. We learned from her that this is how life could be – full of joy and warmth.

Near Death Experience

Martha's story starts with humor too. She came to our group session after weeks of absence. We knew she was critically ill and we had prepared for difficult news. She arrived with a triumphant air. "I've been to the edge of death and back" she declared. While her spirit clearly sparkled, her body told a different story – ravaged by disease, her frame was frail and skeletal and I wondered how she could even stand, let alone navigate so adroitly on her two canes. But her eyes shone with renewed vitality and she smiled widely as she joked "You know you have a problem when your next of kin and priest walk through your hospital door."

Martha was introduced earlier in the chapter as an example of remarkable fighting spirit. Her determination to live, despite the odds, was so strong that even when she was admitted to hospital, critically ill with her options running out, she refused to believe that there was anything seriously wrong. This is her story, mostly in her own words, from the notes I made during the session.

I was in the hospital because fluid had built up in my lungs and it had to be drained and sealed. I thought the fluid was wastage from my tumor and I was shocked to learn that the fluid meant the cancer was now in my lungs. It hit me like a ton of bricks.

A nurse came in to check on me and she couldn't get a pulse. She sounded the alarm. Everyone seemed in a panic, but I was so lucid, so calm. I was thinking, "I'm healthy. There's nothing wrong with me. You guys are wrong."

Despite the procedure the fluid continued to build up in my lungs. The heart lining now filled too. The doctors told me there was nothing more they could do.

I called my husband and said, "I guess you better come. I guess things are pretty serious here."

As the day progressed, her breathing deteriorated. She had to rely on an oxygen mask, she had no breath of her own. "Did you panic then?" a fellow group member wanted to know.

No. I didn't cry. I didn't panic. I was so lucid, it was amazing. I did my bureaucratic thing – get the kids, get the priest, get the lists of things that need to be done.

The family started to arrive. Her children were pulled out of school. She described some very touching moments as friends and family arrived to say goodbye. She told them what she needed to have in place for her children.

There were lots of tears and that was okay. Everybody prayed over me. One after the other they came through the door. It meant telling them "I'm dying. We've fought this for so long. Now, I'm a leaking ship."

She spoke with the priest about funeral arrangements and told him "the hymns I really like." She chose the pall bearers for her funeral, the flowers she would like and what the family should wear.

I was not doubting I was dying. This is it. It's likely today. I'm not going to make it through the night.

Telling her children was the hardest. I was told more than once here in the group, "Maybe you're not letting your kids into your illness." That was so true. Now, I had to admit I was ill. I had to admit I was dying."

Her son lay down on the bed beside her and said "I'm not leaving you. I'm staying here with you. He told her how much he loved her, what a great mother she was. "It was very, moving. He said to me, "If you die, you're going to miss my graduation." She replied, "I know I can't come to your graduation, but I see you're going to be a success."

Her daughter supported her in a way Martha recognized – her daughter was just like herself. "Mom, you're going to be fine. Everything will be alright. You'll come through this. You'll beat this thing."

She was determined not to die until her brother arrived from the other side of the country. She spent the night with her family remembering family times at the cottage. She pantomimed for the group what it was like to drink Tim Hortons coffee together at 4 a.m.: Martha taking a sip, gasping, then grabbing the mask and sucking air, then repeating the process for the next sip. She laughed, enjoying the black humor. When a nurse urged family members to go home so Martha could rest, Martha replied "If I have only 24 hours left to live, I don't want to spend them sleeping."

She had time alone with her husband "talking about the most wonderful things and most mundane things." He asked whether they should still go away on the family vacation they planned, she answered "yes."

She and her family spent time praying. She prayed to die in peace and for her family to be cared for. She did a lot of "rote" praying with her rosary as well. When her brother arrived, Martha said she was ready to die. "I can go now. I feel what I've been praying for. I feel peaceful. I feel accepting. I see all these people around me. It's okay. My children are going to be okay. We're going to be okay. I have had a blessed life."

As soon as she reported that she was ready to go, she started to breathe more easily. The breathing improved until she no longer needed the mask. She had been given steroids and suddenly "they kicked in." But she doesn't believe it was the steroids:

It was the love and prayer I had around me. The power of that. I prayed a lot. If I had died when I first entered the hospital, it would have been shambles. Instead I had this time – to say goodbye to loved ones, to hear what I meant to them, to have their prayers. I went to the edge. I was ready. I can't tell you how calm I was.

The final triumph came the next day when she picked up the phone, called her priest and cancelled her funeral.

We asked her what message she took away from this experience.

For me, the message is about the power of love and relationships. The richness of my life is all about relationships. Also, we don't need to worry. All those things we worry about: Will I die in the hospital or home? Who will be there? All those things take care of themselves. I don't need to control things so much. There was such peace that came with giving over, with surrender. I had such a sense of calm, of knowing my kids would be okay, it was all okay and this calm took away the fear. I was ready and I was calm.

A month later, we asked how the experience had changed her.

It opened the door for people to be more comfortable expressing feelings around dying. The kids retreat back into everyday life now that crisis is over and I think that's good. My husband and I talk more openly about death now.

I've learned I need to let go of always controlling things and acknowledge what others can do. Accept it'll be okay. I realize how silly it is insisting on lists and things being done a certain way. It took going to the brink of death to figure it out. Once you know everything's going to be okay, the rest is bonus.

Later she joked about what her family is likely to do with all her lists after she is gone: she did a ripping pantomime with her hands and laughed heartedly. Martha lived long past the span doctors predicted for her. She made a point of enjoying this "bonus" time with family and friends. She lived with greater openness and acceptance of her situation and strongly felt her life had meaning and direction. She no longer feared dying.

This chapter started with Jake's revelation that "we all have a death sentence" and once we recognize that we can live our lives fully and with meaning. We can live because we want to live, not because we fear dying. This book also speaks to the healing power of warm-hearted connection through the diverse voices and stories of cancer patients and their family members and friends. The book now ends with a story of my own. I believe it weaves together the central themes developed here and serves as a fitting bookend to the wise words of the Dalai Lama which opened this text: "the single most important thing you can do for healing is to cultivate a warm heart."

My Cousin Michael

My cousin Michael was born special. We grew up together in a band of siblings and cousins. Others saw him as different – behind in standard measures of development. We saw that too, but we always knew that he was way ahead of us in other ways. He had huge spirit and heart, always generous and accepting. He had a knack for happiness. He brought it with him wherever he went and within minutes of being in his company, you felt a little lighter, a little happier too. As kids, we valued it. As adults, we came to admire it all the more. We recognized his "difference" for the gift it was, and envied his huge capacity to live his life with fresh enthusiasm every day for all the things he loved – an endless list which included his family and friends, fishing, gardening and local sports teams.

Michael got cancer in his mid thirties: a serious melanoma that had spread to some lymph nodes. It shocked us all. As my cousin David said, "He is the glue of our family." He held and brought us together in so many ways, we couldn't imagine anything bad happening to him. Somehow Michael's difference made him seem exempt from things that could beset others. It was typical of Michael that he remained optimistic and happy throughout his first bout of cancer. Surgery removed the melanoma from his leg and in Michael's mind, it was gone. He did not trouble himself with any thoughts about recurrence even though he knew it could happen. He had so many things that interested him. His innate happiness and enthusiasm for all things continued unabated, whether it was gardening, fishing or going on the family baseball junket. Often Michael's exuberance would pour into a song that he would make-up and sing on the spot, sometimes accompanied with a jig, delightfully oblivious to the odd stares from bystanders. His brothers and cousins, all now married with children, had produced another generation of nephews and nieces who all adored him. More than ever, he was "our glue."

Shortly after his 50th birthday, the melanoma returned as a large incurable mass in his stomach area. There was no standard treatment available likely to make any difference. His brothers searched out experimental trials and found one that promised some hope. It meant a series of very aggressive chemos and an in-hospital stay of a week, each time it was administered.

Michael was never alone. While he was in treatment, some family members stayed for the full time, while others visited in shifts. Michael always went into these treatments upbeat, but the grueling nature of the chemo soon took effect. Mid week was particularly tough, as Michael suffered from extensive vomiting and diarrhea. He was frail, pale and haggard and looked death-ly ill, but he still enjoyed a good joke and was pleased when peo-ple visited. We felt frightened, helpless and saddened by his ordeal. He was so uncomfortable, that it was always a relief when he was able to sleep. One evening I was there when my brother, Doug, arrived from some distance away. Michael was asleep and naturally we did not wake him up.

I hadn't seen Doug for a while and we whispered to each other across Michael's bedside. Around 10 pm, it was time to leave for our hotel. As we got up, Michael's eyes opened and he began to rouse himself. "No," we insisted, "don't wake up," but he did – pulling himself up with some difficulty and evident dis-comfort. It was clear he wanted to say something. It seemed urgent. We could see his determination through his discomfort. Perhaps he needed water or medication? Many hours had gone by. Perhaps he needed us to find a nurse? We leaned over. He whispered. "Thank you for coming. I'm glad you're here." And then he settled back and closed his eyes. Doug and I left the room quietly. I don't think I had ever seen my older brother cry before. Michael's thank you had literally moved him to tears.

It had taken Michael huge effort to rouse himself to speak. And what was it he so urgently needed to say "thank you," an expression of gratitude. His big heart shone through even when he could barely move or speak. We had come to help Michael, but in a strange way, yet again, it was Michael who was helping us: he helped us to see that there is something beyond the needles and the vomiting and the diarrhea. Even with suffering, or perhaps, because of suffering, there is room for this transcendent moment when suffering opens up to something fine and true and lasting: a warm heart and true spirit. This moment is hard to put in words. Body, mind and spirit expand into something larger – call it gratitude; call it love; call it warm-heartedness, call it soul. Whatever it is, there is no doubting its transformative power. Ten years later, my brother and I can recall that moment and feel its undiminished effect. Michael is with us in so many ways.

On the weekend he died, Michael was out fishing with friends. The toll of disease was evident in his frail body, even though he never appeared to take much notice of it. His mind and spirit continued to be strong and he lived fully right till the end. He started bleeding and his fishing buddies took him to the hospital with Michael protesting all the way – he wanted to ignore the bleeding and to continue fishing!

At the hospital Michael underwent emergency surgery to stop the bleeding. The doctor who operated was startled by what he found. The cancer was so extensive he did not know how Michael was even living, let alone out of bed and fishing! He went into a coma and died a day later with all of us, his band of brothers and cousins, at his bedside.

As a family, we were stunned by his loss. There was no one quite like him and even now, nine years later, it is hard to imagine our family without him. Every year on the anniversary of his death, his band of brothers and cousins, nieces and nephews, get together for a celebratory lunch to tell Michael stories. Every year, in the last weekend of June, four generations of our large extended family gather at a lakeside cottage to hold a fishing tournament in his honor. He is still very much "our glue." His big heart and generous spirit live on.

Other Stories

As I end this book with these stories of strong spirit and warm-hearted connection, I am aware they do not speak to everyone. Never far from my mind is the picture of Christine, described in chapter four, isolated and alone, orbiting the earth in a rocketship, far removed from the warmth of human connection, hugging a TV set for companionship. Her story speaks for many too.

It is hard to read stories of human spirit and connection when we feel our life and circumstances are far removed from them. We don't see ourselves in this picture. Remember the central tenet of this book is that from any point, there is always the possibility of moving toward greater comfort and peace. There is a place of opening from wherever you are – whether you are feeling alone, scared and abandoned or whether you are feeling connected, embraced and supported. Much of our suffering comes from believing things should be different than they are. If your circumstances seem bleak, accept that this is the way it is right now. Ask yourself, is there any way you might bring warmth and comfort to yourself in this moment? Perhaps it will be as simple as taking a deep breath and giving yourself some space from this distress. One small step toward greater comfort and peace, brings the next one. Practice the techniques that resonate with you. Find the voices in this book that speak to how you are feeling right now. It is always good to know you are not alone. Don't give up. There are always ways you can help yourself. Let the full range of voices, expressed in these pages, from distress to peace, be your guide. As one moment unfolds into the next, choose to let go of strife and move toward a calm mind and a warm heart.

Notes

Chapter 2

For more information and guidance on managing thoughts:

Burns, D. B. (1999). *Feeling Good Handbook.* New York: Plume.

Chapter 3

Breath Awareness:

Hanh, Thich Nhat. (2003).*Creating True Peace.* New York, Free Press.

Relaxation:

Benson, Herbert. (1975). *The Relaxation Response.* New York: William Morrow.

Benson, Herbert. (1996). *Timeless Healing.* New York: Scribner.

Meditation:

Bodian, Stephen. (2006). *Meditation for Dummies.* Hoboken, NJ: Wiley.

Davidson, R.J., Kabat-Zinn, J, Shumacher, J., Rosenkranz, M., Muller, D., Santorelli, S.F., Urbanowski, F. and Harrington, A. (2003) Alterations in brain and immune function produced by mindfulness meditation. *Psychosomatic Medicine, 65,*: 564-570.

Hölzel, B.K., Carmody, J., Vangel, M., Congleton, C., Yerramsetti, S.M., Gard, T., and Lazar, S.W. (2011). Mindfulness practice leads to increases in regional brain gray matter density. *Psychiatry Research: Neuroimaging,; 191* (1): 36-43.

Kabat-Zinn, J., Lipworth, L., and Burney, R. (1985). The clinical use of mindfulness meditations for the regulation of chronic pain. *Journal of Behavioral Medicine, 8,*: 163-190.

Kabat-Zinn, J. (1990).Full *Catastrophic Living: Using the Wisdom of Your Body and Mind to Face Stress, Pain and Illness.* New York, Delacorte.

Kabat-Zinn, J, Massion, A.O., Kristeller, J, Peterson, L.G., Fletcher, K.E., Pbert, L., Lenderking, W.R., Santorelli, S.F. (1992). Effectiveness of a meditation-based stress reduction program in the treatment of anxiety disorders. *Am J Psych 149*:936–43.

Meares, A. (1980). What can the cancer patient expect from intensive meditation? *Australian Family Physician, 9*, 322-324.

Guided Imagery:

Archterberg, J. (1985). *Imagery in Healing: Shamanism and Modern Medicine.* Boston: Shambhala.

Edmonds, C.V.I., Phillips, C., & Cunningham, A.J.C. (2001). The focused mind: Using hypnosis, relaxation, guided imagery and meditation to help cancer patients cope. In Jennifer Baraclough (ed.) *Complementary Cancer Care: Towards Integration?* Oxford: Oxford Press.

Eremin O, Walker, MB, Simpson, E., Heys, S.D., Ah-See, A.K., Hutcheon, A.W., Ogston, K.N., Sarkar, T.K., Segar, A., Walker, L.G.(2009). Immuno-modulatory effects of relaxation training and guided imagery in women with locally advanced breast cancer undergoing multimodality therapy: a randomised controlled trial. *Breast. Feb;18*(1):17-25.

Rossman, M.L. (2000). Guided Imagery for Self-healing. Tiburon, CA: Kramer.

Journaling:

DeSalvo, L. (2000). Writing as a Way of Healing. Boston: Beacon Press.

Pennebaker, J.W. (1990). *Opening up: The Healing Power of Expressing Emotions.* New York: Guilford Press.

Pennebaker, J.W. & Beall, S K. (1986) Confronting a traumatic event. Toward an understanding of inhibition and disease. *Journal of Abnormal Psychology, 95*, 274–281

Smyth, J.M., Stone, A.A., Hurewitz, A., & Kaell, A. (1999). Effects of writing about stressful experiences on symptom reduction in patients with asthma or rheumatoid arthritis: A randomized trial. *JAMA, 281*, 1304-1309.

Chapter 4

Social Support and Recovery:

Anthony, W.A. (1993). Recovery from mental illness: the guiding vision of the mental health service system in the 1990s. *Psychosocial Rehabilitation Journal, 16* (4) 11-23.

Barth, J., Schneider, S., and von Känel, R. (2010). Lack of social support in the etiology and the prognosis of coronary heart disease: A systematic review and meta-analysis. *Psychosomatic Medicine, 72:* 229-238

House, J.S.K., Landis, R., and Umberson, D. (1988). Social relationships and health, *Science,241*:540-45.

Umberson, D. and Montez, J.K. (2010). Social relationships and health. *Journal of Health and Social Behavior 1* : S54-S66.

Spiegel, D. (2011). Mind matters in cancer survival. *JAMA, 305*(5):502-503.

Chapter 5

Goleman, D. (2003). *Destructive Emotions: How can we overcome them?* New York: Bantam. See chapter 1, "The lama in the lab" for a description of Davidson's work with Tibetan monks.

Davidson, R.J., Kabat-Zinn, J, Shumacher, J., Rosenkranz, M., Muller, D., Santorelli, S.F., Urbanowski, F.,and Harrington, A. (2003) Alterations in brain and immune function produced by mindfulness meditation. *Psychosomatic Medicine,65,:* 564-570.

Luskin, F. (2003). *Forgive for Good.* New York: Harper Collins

Ornish, D. (1990). *Reversing Heart Disease.* NewYork: Ballantine Books.

Ornish, D. (1998). *Love and Survival.* New York: Harper Collins.

Tolle, E. (1997). *The Power of Now.* Vancouver: Namaste

Chapter 6

Forgiveness:

Luskin, F. (2003). *Forgive for Good.* New York: Harper Collins.

Overcoming anger and hurt:

Goleman, D. (2003). *Destructive Emotions: How can we overcome them?* New York: Bantam.

Loving Kindness Meditation:

Kornfield, J. (1993). *A Path with Heart.* New York: Bantam Books. See chapter 1: "Did I love well?"

Cultivating Compassion:

Armstrong, K. (2010). *Twelve Steps to a Compassionate Life.* New York: Knopf

Dalai Lama and Cutler, H.C. (1998). *The Art of Happiness.* New York: Riverhead Books.

Gratitude Journal:

Ben-Shahar, T. (2010). *Even Happier: A Gratitude Journal for Daily and Lasting Fulfillment.* New York: McGraw Hill.

Inner Healer and other guided imagery exercises:

Rossman, M.L. (2000). *Guided Imagery for Self-healing.* Tiburon, CA: Kramer.

Rossman, M.L. (2003). *Fighting Cancer from Within.* New York: Holt.

An inner healer mp3 file is available for download at *www.healing journey.ca.* See audio CDs which complement Levels I and II workbooks and download the level II CD. This link takes you to a cancer resource centre in England.

Healing Light:

Thondup, T. (2000). *Boundless Healing.* Boston: Shambhala

Thondup, T. (1996). *The Healing Power of Mind.* Boston: Shambhala

Radha, Swami S. (1987). *The Divine Light Invocation.* Spokane: Timeless books.

Chapter 8:

Cunningham, A.J. (2005). *Can the Mind Heal Cancer? A Clinician-Scientist Examines the Evidence.*

Cunningham, A.J. and Watson, K. (2004). How psychological therapy may prolong survival in cancer patients: New evidence and a simple theory. *Integrative Cancer Therapies (3)*: 214-229.

Cunningham, A.S., Phillips, C., Lockwood, G.A., Hedley, D. and Edmonds, C.U.I. (2000). Association of involvement in psychological self help with longer survival in patients with metastatic cancer: An exploratory study. *Advances in Mind-Body Medicine, 16,* 276-294

Cunningham, A.J., Edmonds, C.U.I., Phillips, C., Soots, K.I., Hedley, D. and Lockwood, G.A. (2000). A prospective longitudinal study of the relationship of psychological work and duration of survival in patients with metastatic cancer. *Psycho-oncology, 9*: 323-339.

Tolle, E. (1997). *The Power of Now.* Vancouver: Namaste

Albom, M. (2002). *Tuesdays with Morrie.* New York: Random House.

The quote from John Cleese's memorial for Graham Chapman was first brought to my attention by the CBC radio program, Tapestry. The program, "Death, be not scary" aired on April 17, 2011 and focused on the role of humor and spirit in dealing with death. Tapestry, a weekly program, is an excellent resource for exploring issues related to spirituality and meaning. See http://www.cbc.ca/tapestry/episode/2011/04/17/death-be-not-scary/